Behind the Smile

The mouth tells a story that shapes your child's future

Dr Donny Mandrawa

'Dr Donny Mandrawa and I share a vision of early functional guidance for families - particularly those with children on the autism spectrum. His book *Behind the Smile* beautifully reflects this shared purpose. Through Ethan's story, Dr Donny shows how structures and functions can change with time and care - and how bodywork, myofunctional therapy, and dental treatment can bring about profound improvements.

'He encourages parents to trust their instincts, seek early intervention, and build the right multidisciplinary team. Like Dr Donny, I view parents and children as central members of that team. His holistic approach - combining dental, neurological, and functional perspectives - helps families understand that growth and healing come from collaboration.

'Dr Donny also explains how early development shapes lifelong function. Mouth and airway growth begin in utero, with reflexes and feeding experiences guiding future speech and breathing. He reminds us that chewing strengthens facial muscles and bones, and that good movement, feeding, and posture support healthy oral and airway development.

'*Behind the Smile* brings together science, clinical insight, and compassion - an inspiring reminder that when parents, practitioners, and children work together, extraordinary progress is possible.'

Diane Bahr MS, *CCC-SLP, CIMI*
Speech-Language Pathologist, Infant Massage Instructor, Author, International Speaker
Las Vegas, US

'Dr Donny is having an amazing impact in the world with his wonderful ability to connect with people and share his passion and knowledge around all things Oral-facial function, growth, and development. He is a dentist by training, but he does not look just at the teeth - he looks at the human being that those teeth are connected to and allows the teeth to tell him a story.

'His collaborative approach to the health of the individual is what sets him apart and is why he has been so successful in practice - leading his team with this patient-centric care approach. He has a following as an educator in the field and has trained and inspired many other practitioners in this holistic approach... both from within the dental field and outside.

‘I am excited to read this new book by Dr Donny where he shares the health journey of a child and their family – providing hope and inspiration for families, empowering them to take control of their health and see what can be done when working with the support of a team of amazing clinicians.

‘We need more clinicians like Dr Donny in the world – who are looking at the health potential of the child in front of them and who can “open the doors and turn on the lights” and allow a dimmed life expression to become a vibrant picture of health.’

Dr Mary Bourke *BSc (Anat) BAppSc (Chiro)*
Chiropractor, CEO and Clinical Advisor of Myo Munchee
Newcastle, Australia

‘My daughter was born with achondroplasia (Dwarfism) and, at just 13 months old, was diagnosed with severe obstructive sleep apnea. The only option we were given was a CPAP, which felt like a short-term fix – not a long-term solution.

‘After sharing my concerns with our chiropractor, he recommended Dr Donny. That conversation changed everything.

‘With Dr Donny’s guidance, we followed an innovative approach that addressed the root causes. Today, my daughter is nine, thriving, and no longer needs her CPAP. Her sleep apnea is now classified as mild – something we once thought impossible.

‘We are incredibly grateful to Dr Donny for his extensive knowledge, which has allowed our daughter the chance to breathe, grow, and live more freely.’

Cassandra

‘I used to suffer from a wide range of difficulties – difficulty articulating my words properly, difficulty breathing, and incessant headaches throughout the entire day. In some cases, I wouldn’t be able to string together a coherent sentence due to compromised speech patterns. Although I wasn’t rendered completely dysfunctional, these difficulties turned what most people found gratification in doing into a blur drowned in a noise of discomfort; it made it difficult to truly enjoy anything.

'When I was 10 years old, I started myofunctional treatment and a tongue tie correction with Dr Donny Mandrawa and his team, which helped to alleviate many of these difficulties. Already within three years of commitment, I could enjoy activities (like running) without being assaulted by intense headaches. It became far easier to communicate due to improved speech patterns, and my daily endeavors weren't constantly interrupted by congestion; life was no longer drowned in constant discomfort nearly as much. I'm grateful that I had the opportunity to undergo this treatment; otherwise, I would've continued to suffer from these difficulties up until today.'

James

'I met Donny Mandrawa in 2019 in Australia while I was visiting to teach a pediatric sleep course. I visited his clinic, saw his work, and reviewed his treatment protocols, and I was instantly fascinated by his approach to pediatric airways. Over time, through several discussions and exchanges of ideas about airway health in children, I can say that I have met someone who is very passionate about the holistic evaluation and management of pediatric airways through myofunctional therapy. We have taught courses together, and I can say that Donny is a great teacher and fun to learn from.

'Myofunctional therapy has recently emerged as one of the critical interventions in the management of pediatric airway-related sleep disorders such as snoring, mouth breathing, and obstructive sleep apnea. Interacting with Donny, it has become very clear to me that early diagnosis and early intervention with such therapies are the cornerstones of optimizing airway health and improving functional outcomes of several dental and surgical interventions for pediatric sleep-disordered breathing. This is the critical intervention that can correct the form, function, and stability of the airways.

'In a world where children's developmental challenges are too often treated in isolation, *Behind The Smile* is a clarion call for holistic thinking and early intervention. Dr Mandrawa writes this book from the rare vantage point of an experienced myofunctional dentist who has also lived through the sleepless nights and limited choices of a parent. He clearly explains how everyday functional issues (from breastfeeding struggles and tongue-tie to snoring, attention problems, and narrow jaws) are interconnected, why multidisciplinary teamwork matters, and how families can move from confusion to competent action. The story of Ethan is both a comforting companion for worried parents and a practical case study for practitioners. This book doesn't just inform – it empowers you to understand the underlying fundamentals of health and wellbeing. It is highly recommended for parents, pediatricians, dentists, speech therapists, and anyone committed to improving children's long-term health and overall potential. This book is an indispensable resource for professionals and parents who are dedicated to guiding children towards achieving thriving futures.'

Dr Umakanth Katwa *MD*
Pediatric Pulmonologist & Sleep Medicine Specialist,
Assistant Professor of Pediatrics Boston Children's Hospital,
Harvard Medical School
Boston, US

'I have had the privilege of knowing Dr Donny Mandrawa for many years, both as a colleague and as a close friend, and I can say without hesitation that he is one of the most impressive and inspiring clinicians I have ever met. Donny is a born leader, someone who naturally brings out the best in those around him. He has built an incredible team of passionate and dedicated professionals who share his vision of putting patients' wellbeing first. It is immediately apparent, whether you step into his practice or listen to one of his lectures, that the culture he has created is one grounded in care, respect, and excellence.

'What sets Donny apart is his rare combination of clinical precision, emotional intelligence, and genuine compassion. He treats every patient as an individual, understanding that each person's journey is unique. He takes the time to consider every aspect of a patient's life, not only their dental or facial concerns but also their readiness for treatment, family dynamics, and even their genetic background. He believes that true orthodontic care involves looking beyond the surface and understanding the story that has led the patient to where they are. His ability to see the bigger picture and tailor his treatment accordingly is what makes his work so profoundly impactful.

'Donny is also a forward thinker in every sense. He constantly challenges the boundaries of traditional orthodontics, integrating the latest research and technology into his practice while maintaining a deep respect for the fundamentals of evidence-based care. His philosophy is one of early, gentle, and balanced intervention, always seeking to guide growth and function rather than force change. He embodies the integrative and collaborative approach that I believe represents the future of healthcare. His work brings together the expertise of multiple disciplines to ensure that every patient receives holistic, comprehensive care.

'As an educator, Donny is equally exceptional. He has a wealth of evidence-based knowledge, and his presenting style is full of energy, authenticity, and humor. Whether he is speaking to students, practitioners, or parents, he has a gift for turning complex ideas into engaging, accessible insights. He inspires others not only through his words but through the consistency of his actions and the integrity of his practice.

'It is about time that he has written a book, and frankly, it is long overdue. Donny has so much wisdom to share, and his unique blend of clinical expertise and human insight will undoubtedly make this work both inspirational and transformative. I have no doubt that it will benefit parents, health practitioners, and educators alike. His contribution to our profession continues to raise standards and touch lives, and I am proud to call him both a colleague and a friend.'

Dr Derek Mahony *BDS (Syd), MScOrth (Lon), DOrthRCS (Edin), MDOrthRCPS (Glas), MOrthRCS (Eng), FRCD (Can), MOrth RCS (Edin), FICD, IBO, FACD, FICCDE, FIADFE, FPFA, Grad Dip Dental Sleep Medicine (UWA), FCGDent, Grad Dip Ortho (Lon), FDSM, MBA (Wharton), FDS RCS(Eng), Grad Dip Dental Sleep Medicine (Lon), MSc Clear Aligner Therapy (Lon)*
Specialist Airway Orthodontist, International Speaker
Sydney, Australia

‘Firstly, I wanted to say that nothing I write will ever show my gratitude towards Donny. Dr Donny is one of the most humble, honest people and dentists you will ever meet. We are still in awe of the difference your treatment plan made without any surgery or extractions, which was our goal from the start. I will always recommend Dr Donny to everyone I meet because I know from experience with my son Matthew that it isn’t about the money; it’s always about the outcome for the patient he treats.

‘Thank you again from the bottom of our hearts. We are still in awe of Dr Donny’s work and intelligence.’

Marleine

‘Dr Donny has created an easy-reading, yet comprehensive gem in this book. Each parent will want to read it before they embark, and refer to it often as they and their child navigate the world of optimal health through nature-based functional dental orthopedics.

‘Written from the perspective of a deeply caring parent and eyes-wide-open professional who has experienced firsthand the challenges of guiding his own children through this often (and increasingly) complex process, Dr Donny is able to bridge the chasm between hard science and the practicalities of everyday life. He makes it both understandable and individually applicable.

‘The transformation that so naturally unfolds as the patient is thus empowered to become an active and key participant in their treatment is magical to behold. This book gives you many of the critical instructions that we wish all kids came with.’

Dr Darick Nordstrom *DDS*
Inventor of ALF Therapy, Holistic Orthodontic Pioneer
San Diego, US

'I met Dr Mandrawa in 2024 in Australia and Japan during my courses on fascia and the osteopathic approach to the stomatognathic system. Through our many conversations, I was pleased to finally meet a professional who recognized so many similarities between osteopathic principles and myofunctional therapy.

'Recent evidence shows that myofunctional therapy is a critical intervention in pediatric dentistry, especially for sleep-disordered breathing and non-nutritive sucking habits, and their impact on growth and development. As an osteopath, I believe collaboration between our professions can be extremely fruitful for young patients.

'We share the same belief in early, individualized intervention. Acting early can prevent issues such as crowded teeth, speech impediments, tongue thrust and sleep-disordered breathing, reducing the need for complex treatments later in life.

'Dr Mandrawa's approach mirrors osteopathic principles: personalized exercises to retrain oral and facial muscles, improve function, and establish correct oral posture to support healthy breathing, jaw and dental development. His commitment to transdisciplinary teamwork and holistic care continues to inspire me.'

Dr Paolo Tozzi *MSc Ost, BSc (Hons) Ost*
DO Osteopath, Physiotherapist, TSRM member, Posturologist,
Reiki Master
Rome, Italy

To David,
who is shining down upon us

First published in 2026 by Dr Donny Mandrawa

A catalogue entry for this book is available from the National Library of Australia.

ISBN: 978-1-923630-12-3

Printed in Australia by Pegasus
Book production and text design by Publish Central
Cover design by Pipeline Design

The paper this book is printed on is certified as environmentally friendly.

Disclaimer: The material in this publication is of the nature of general comment only and does not represent professional medical, dental or health advice. It is not intended to provide specific guidance for particular circumstances and should not be relied on as the basis for any decision to take or not take action on any matter it covers. Readers should seek appropriate professional advice from qualified health practitioners before making any decisions about diagnosis, treatment or care. To the maximum extent permitted by law, the author and publisher disclaim all responsibility and liability to any person arising directly or indirectly from any person taking or not taking action based on the information in this publication.

While this book is based on real events, certain details, timelines and conversations have been adapted or dramatised for narrative purposes. Not every element represents an exact account of actual events or dialogue.

Contents

Introduction: why parents need to read this book

The long and narrow road

Many families have been on long journeys, trying to find answers and resolutions for the issues their children face. I am referring to functional issues that impact the natural growth and development of these children. Issues such as the inability to breastfeed, difficulty swallowing, delayed speech development, mouth breathing, snoring, poor sleep, being constantly tired, lack of focus and concentration, sudden tantrums, defiance, and hyperactivity – to name just a few.

In my almost 30 years of practicing dentistry, I have never seen such an explosion of functional issues as that which has occurred in the last 15 or so years. Is this because more people are becoming better educated to assess, detect, and recognize them? Or is it because our society is changing so rapidly that these issues are becoming more prevalent?

Whatever the reasons are, I believe that our children are growing up in a dangerous time. Too many of them are facing developmental problems, resulting in significant challenges for parents to navigate. The most challenging aspect of it is actually trying to find health providers who understand what they are going through and are able to formulate a plan that guides and helps them reach a positive outcome – basically, being the 'directors' of these families to continue to move forward.

Been there, done that

When my wife and I had our first child in 2007, we experienced firsthand the challenges that a lot of the families I now see are going through. Our firstborn had a tongue tie, and our second also had one.

The oldest would wake up every 40 minutes throughout the night, and my wife told me to sleep in the guest bedroom so that I could be well-rested for the safety of the patients I would see the next day. (Yes, I accidentally poked a patient on the lower lip with a sharp instrument once because I was sleep-deprived from a crying baby waking me up constantly the night before.)

And with the youngest, breastfeeding was a struggle. I still remember being awake all night before we had to catch an early-morning flight for a family trip, as my wife had mastitis and was in excruciating pain. She spent the entire night with her in the bathtub, with us trying everything to relieve the discomfort. I was ready to cancel our entire trip by sunrise, but we decided to push through with the holiday. Well, as you can imagine, we did absolutely nothing and stayed in our hotel room during that break as we were completely exhausted.

Two types of health providers

There are two types of health providers out there. One is stuck in their ways, trapping themselves in a box, keeping their minds on the same narrow path. The other type are free thinkers who believe in continuous learning, not only from their own profession but from others as well, because they usually question the *why*. The latter tend to keep their minds open to concepts and philosophies that may seem foreign to them initially, but they are willing to explore and study them more.

The free thinkers understand that the body is made up of various functioning systems that are interconnected, and so they strive to find the root causes of problems. Thinking that each system works independently fails to appreciate the complexity of how a body functions. Sure, it is much easier to just understand one than to understand many. It is also much easier to assess and treat one, thinking that other issues are not related.

If teeth are crowded and have no space, would you see a dentist who evaluates the causes of the crowded teeth and addresses the reasons behind the problem, or would you see a dentist who just looks at and treats the teeth only, without even finding out the cause? If you choose the former, your dentist is likely to be a free thinker, and I can almost guarantee that this dentist works in a collaborative manner alongside other health providers.

Having that team approach is an important part of healthcare. Each provider has their own scope of practice, which needs to be respected and followed. However, all systems in the body are linked, where one problem in one system may arise from and/or lead to a problem in another system. Every provider needs other providers to solve the jigsaw puzzle as well as they can.

No one can work alone.

This book may give the answer

This, in turn, brings on other challenges for these families. Which type of providers do we have to see? Who do we see first? How many of them do we have to see? How long is this going to take? What happens if we are not able to follow the plan? Does that mean I am a bad parent?

With this book, I hope that I will be able to answer all of those questions, providing a clear direction for families to make their journeys more achievable.

I set my mission many years ago when my firstborn arrived. I traveled down the long winding road myself, often alone as a family, and often lost, where every corner seemed to be a wrong turn. We managed to climb over many hills and mountains to get to where we are now. I pursued countless studies to equip myself with vast knowledge, which opened the door for me to hone my skill-set while integrating my care in a collaborative environment. The easier path did not interest me. I felt and still feel the importance of facing these threats head-on.

Having been to many parts of the world, I have come to realize that the problem is universal, affecting those growing up in modern societies. Similar patterns keep surfacing from one country to another. The world is evolving at an unprecedented rate. Who would've guessed 20 years ago that there would be a medical condition called 'tech neck' or 'text neck syndrome'? How are all the technological developments affecting the ways our children grow? From the food we eat to the air we breathe, modern conveniences are taking human beings further away from nature.

Read Ethan's story from start to finish

I will take you on a brief journey about a boy named Ethan and how, as a team, we navigated the obstacles and barriers to help him reach his destination.[1] His tale is one of courage, patience, and faith. One that needs to be followed from beginning to the end. My hope is for you, the parents out there, to take note and learn about the warning signs your children may have, which may be indicative of the need to intervene early. You must understand the measures to take and the doors to open. Take note of the elements and the options to consider. Take note of what is required to uncover hidden, unique genetic potentials.

This is not fiction but a step-by-step recount of a true story. A retelling based on one journey that revealed much more than the eyes could see. Pay attention to the details embedded inside each paragraph. Pause after each chapter and take your time to think about the similarities that your children (and maybe yourself) may have with Ethan's story. I invite you to immerse yourself in the experience from start to finish and see how much it resonates with what you are going through.

Many of you may have a child like Ethan – a child who is strong and resilient but struggling and vulnerable under the surface. In fact, maybe all of our children are similar. They are good at hiding behind their own walls. Not because they are afraid, but because they need to protect themselves from the unknown.

So, is it our role to set them free to grow and flourish in health? This may sound cliché, but our children truly are our future. And so, my mission is to play my part in optimizing functional health for the sake of future generations. No matter how small that part is ...

---

1 Ethan and Sally are based on real patients under my care; however, their names and identifying details have been changed to protect their privacy and maintain confidentiality.

1

Enter Ethan

The child who wasn't seen

I never knew Ethan existed until his mother brought him in to see me on a late winter afternoon. He was quiet and would not make eye contact when we first met. There was a strong sense of awkwardness. He did not know where to look, and neither did I, not wanting to stare at him to make him uncomfortable.

He sat in the chair in the middle of the room when I invited him to. Clearly he understood me, but not a word came out of his mouth. Sally, his mother, did all the talking. 'He is 10 already, and I didn't think you would be interested in seeing him,' she said. I could sense the desperation in her, sounding helpless and lost, with only a small glimmer of hope in her eyes.

My heart was pounding as a surge of intense anxiety came over me. How could I not know about this boy? I had known his older brother for two years by then, and I had no clue that there was a younger one! Well, he was now sitting right in front of me, and despite feeling uneasy, I felt the need to get to know him more. Not because I felt obligated to do so, but because I wanted to. There was something peculiar about him that I wanted to uncover. And so I remained curious.

Questions began racing through my head. What was his mother expecting of me? Why had she never told me about him? Whenever his older brother came to see me, how come he never came along? Why was he never even mentioned before? Why suddenly now did his mother think it would be the right time? Why, why, why ...

'So, what is the reason you've brought him to see me today?' I asked his mother with a slight tremble in my voice. I didn't know if I was good enough at hiding my look of surprise. I became self-conscious about how I was sitting in front of them. Should I cross my legs? Should I fold my arms? Should I hide behind my imaginary desk?

'Well, no one wants to help him. I've taken him to see many others, and all of them told us to just wait. After seeing the incredible results you managed to achieve with my older one, I thought I'd bring Ethan now to see if you could help him,' she answered. 'Everyone else I had taken him to told me to come back when he's much older, as there's nothing they could do now,' she continued.

I put on my confident front, deepening my tone, slowing down my pace, and opening my stance to show them both that I am here ... you are safe ... I am welcoming you both with open arms and an open mind.

It was very obvious they were seeking a place of comfort, where they would both feel secure and, more importantly, accepted.

A similar case: what early intervention can achieve

The day Ethan came, I had just completed another of my patient's early intervention treatments that afternoon. She had initially been referred to me by her neurodevelopmental chiropractor because she had been turned away by several orthodontists. They all told her to come back when she was older, as she was 'too young to have anything done'.

'Well, Sally, funny you should bring him in today,' I said. 'I have just completed treatment on a 10-year-old girl, the same age as Ethan. Her teeth were crowded, her jaws were narrow, and her bite was deep,' I shared with her. Sally's eyes widened as she took in this coincidence. I continued, 'When I first met her, she had seen a few orthodontists, and they all told her the same thing: wait until she's older.'

This patient was seeing her pediatric dentist every six months. The dentist would check the health of her teeth and gums, but never evaluated how she was functioning. She was dysfunctionally breathing through her mouth.

Mouth breathing means the tongue needs to sit low to allow a passage for air to go in and out. The tongue, however, is the best expander of the upper jaw. When it sits and places forces up against the roof of the mouth, or the palate, the upper jaw widens. This jaw houses the upper teeth, and so, consequently, the upper teeth then have more space to erupt into better alignment. Additionally, because the tongue has shaped the upper jaw, this also means the tongue has sufficient room to be housed up in the palate.

The lower jaw sits under the upper jaw. This is the jaw that is more mobile, as it can open and close, as well as move side to side, to facilitate various functions. The lower teeth sit in the lower jaw. Because this jaw is positioned under the upper, its growth tends to be determined and guided by the upper jaw. A wider upper jaw usually leads to a wider lower jaw.

I explained to Sally and Ethan, 'For her, it took us 10 months of exercise-based treatment. My orofacial myofunctional therapist and I prescribed various exercises for the muscles of her mouth and face. The aims were to improve her tongue posture, tongue strength, lip closure, and breathing habits. She was also continuing to receive adjustments from her chiropractor. Because the functions of her mouth and face improved, her jaws began to develop in the right direction. Her teeth and bite then followed.' Ethan continued to look up toward the corner of the room, as Sally's face began to beam with anticipation.

By the end of her active treatment, my patient's dysfunctional breathing had been corrected. Her jaws were wide and able to accommodate her existing and future teeth. There was plenty of room for her tongue to sit right up against the palate. Not only was she in a much better position structurally, but also functionally.

Her treatment outcomes were achieved because she still had growth potential. The jaws are part of the bones of the face and head, or the cranium. The face has completed 60% of natural growth by the age of four years, 80% by six, and 90% between nine and eleven. This is one reason why I prefer to intervene early.

'But Sally,' I added, 'everyone is different. I hope I will be able to help Ethan.' Sally understood that I was trying not to promise anything. She smiled with approval.

Look beyond the structures

I come across many families that have been told the same story over and over again: wait until the patient is older, until they have no more baby teeth. Then let's extract some teeth to make room so the orthodontic braces can straighten the remaining teeth. They are told it is much easier this way, as the aim is only to have straight teeth.

Ethan was brought to see me because his mother was lost. 'I don't understand why other dentists and orthodontists never asked me these questions about how Ethan is breathing, sleeping, chewing, swallowing, speaking, and behaving, like you did,' Sally exclaimed.

These practitioners are totally ignoring the importance of functions. They just focus on the structures! This is sad, in my opinion. Sad that most health practitioners would rather manage patients via the easiest ways. Yes, the easiest way is to only look at one piece of the jigsaw puzzle instead of looking at how the pieces are actually connected. Is it because they *do not want to know*, or because they simply *do not know*?

Lucky for Ethan, he still had time ...

CHAPTER 1 KEY FINDINGS

- As a parent, trust your instincts if you feel something is not quite right.
- If you have been on a long journey to find answers, don't give up; keep persisting until you've found a practitioner who understands you.
- Intervene as soon as the functional issues are detected.

2

It's all connected

Which came first, the chicken or the egg? It's an old riddle we've all heard, but it's also the perfect way to describe the tangled relationships inside the human body. In oral health, one issue often triggers another, and before long, it's hard to know where the first problem began. Did the mouth breathing start because the nose was blocked, or did the nose become blocked because the mouth was doing all the work? Did the tongue sit low because the jaw was narrow, or did the jaw become narrow because the tongue never sat where it should?

When we see a child like Ethan, we're not just looking for a single cause – we're looking for the chain reaction. Understanding these connections is key to helping a child grow, breathe, and function properly. In this chapter, we'll explore how habits, posture, breathing, and muscle strength influence each other, sometimes in subtle ways that go unnoticed until the signs are obvious.

Why tongue posture matters

As Ethan's appointment went on, I kept noticing that his mouth was constantly open, with his tongue sitting low in his mouth. 'I can see that Ethan's tongue sits on the bottom of his mouth,' I pointed out to Sally. 'It is not exerting forces up against his upper jaw from the inside out. The lips and cheeks are muscles that are always sitting over and against the upper jaw, exerting forces from the outside in. For the upper jaw to widen, the forces from the inside need to be greater than those from the outside. Therefore, the tongue needs to sit up and function against the roof of the mouth.'

Sally replied, 'No one ever explained that to me before. This is the first time I have understood why his teeth are crowded.'

The tongue is one of the strongest muscles in the body. It is the second muscle to be formed, after the heart, when the fetus begins to grow in the womb, demonstrating how important this organ is to human development. It can exert a force of up to 500 grams. To move a lower tooth, only a force of three to four grams is required.

If a person is mouth breathing, has a tongue tie, and/or has low tongue tone, the tongue sits low in the mouth, leading to the jaws being narrowed. However, a narrowed upper jaw also means there is insufficient space for the tongue to fit up against the palate. So then, which one came first, the low tongue or the narrow upper jaw?

When breathing goes wrong

A similar chicken or egg scenario happens with mouth breathing. When the nose, which is made for breathing, is not being utilized sufficiently for its purpose, it becomes more congested due to the lack of air current traveling in and out through it. The congested nose also leads to the need to mouth breathe more.

Mouth breathing also means the air flowing through the mouth does not get filtered or humidified. The tonsils, which are our lymphatic glands and are part of our immune system, need to work harder to protect the body when pathogens enter. When the tonsils enlarge, they narrow the throat. If the tonsils are so large that they obstruct the airway, air cannot get through from the nasal passages, resulting in the need to open the mouth and mouth breathe.

Additionally, when the nervous system is dysregulated, such as when the person is in fight-or-flight mode (sympathetic overdrive), because the body is under stress, there is usually a need to over-breathe. But over-breathing places the body under more stress, resulting in the person being more sympathetically driven.

Ethan was listening to the conversation his mother and I were having. His mouth remained open the entire time. Not once did he close his lips together, except for when he was swallowing every now and then.

I proceeded to show Sally the effects of his open mouth posture. 'You see, when his mouth is constantly open, his cheek muscles are actually exerting more forces inward, narrowing his upper jaw further.' I invited Sally to try this herself. She opened her mouth and could feel the immediate tension of her cheeks against her upper jaw. Her hands were touching her cheeks on both sides as she nodded in agreement.

Comfort sucking and mouth development

Many babies use a pacifier to soothe themselves. It can be an effective method of settling a baby down. However, when the baby sucks on the pacifier, the aberrant forces push the upper jaw up and forward while the lower jaw goes down and back. This leads to the development of an open bite when the teeth begin to erupt, which means the upper and lower front teeth cannot meet and bite together.

Not only are the teeth and jaws affected, but the tongue gets pushed down to the floor of the mouth. The sucking motion also encourages the tongue to thrust forward instead of elevating up toward the palate. Quite different from breastfeeding.

When the baby has a pacifier for too long, the open bite generally worsens, and the tongue thrust becomes habitual. Hence, when use of the pacifier ceases, the tongue tends to continue to thrust forward, partly due to the need for it to seal the gap that is the open bite. This gap creates a problem when speaking, chewing, and swallowing. (My suggestion is to cease the use of a pacifier by six months old.)

The forward tongue thrust continues to push the upper jaw forward, where it becomes pointy and protrusive. As the tongue moves back in after each forward thrust, it brings the lower jaw down and back. Consequently, the open bite may not resolve, even when the pacifier has been eliminated. If these repercussions remain, the child may be at a higher risk of developing breathing dysfunctions, sleep disorders, and possibly needing more significant orthodontic treatment, including jaw surgery.

These effects on the jaws, teeth, and tongue are comparable to those caused by thumb-sucking and finger-sucking habits. They all fall into the category of 'non-nutritive sucking'. Interestingly, I have noticed that babies tend to suck on a pacifier, their thumbs, or their fingers when they have a tongue tie. This makes sense because when the tongue is unable to lift all the way up to the roof of the mouth, the palate does not receive sufficient stimulation to improve sensory processing, calm the nervous system, and enhance the brain–body connection.

But bear in mind that babies who have non-nutritive sucking habits do not always have tongue ties. They may have low tongue posture and low tongue tone but with no restrictions, which again brings forward the question of which causes which to begin with.

A vicious cycle

As you can see, one issue affects another, then another, which in turn affects the first detected issue. It is like a vicious cycle that never ends. And with the examples above, I have only mentioned the tongue and the breathing functions. There are many other systems within the body that are interconnected. Even the tongue and breathing themselves can affect much more.

Digging deeper into the history of each patient with the hope of finding the root causes is the foundation of an effective management plan. Often the root causes are not apparent initially, and so further investigations are needed to eventually get closer to the source. This is where it becomes challenging and usually interesting. The deeper you dig, the more hidden buried treasures you find.

'Can I ask you more questions about Ethan, Sally?' I tried to gain her permission.

'Of course,' she answered. 'I may not know all the answers, but I will give you as much information as I can,' she added.

I felt reassured that we were on the same page. I was trying to gather as much detail as I could, as what had happened to Ethan so far might provide me with clues that could be related to where he ended.

Every child goes through a period of rapid growth and development. This process is highly dynamic and can be influenced by many factors, often without anyone realizing it. When something in the system changes, the body is remarkably quick to adapt to survive. If a child can't breathe properly through the nose, they begin to mouth breathe. The mouth opens, the tongue sits low, and the upper jaw narrows. To keep the airway open, the head tilts forward and the neck muscles tighten. Even swallowing, sleeping, and posture adapt to maintain balance. These are clever short-term solutions – but over time, they mask the real cause.

Consequently, it becomes much more difficult to find the root causes. The adaptive changes end up masking one dysfunction after another, leading to the need to peel the layers of the onion one at a time until the core is uncovered. This peeling of the onion takes time, as the body needs to be given the opportunity and the space to unravel itself before revealing its blueprint.

A collaborative model of care

Because there are so many layers, it's impossible for just one person to do all the peeling. It also helps to share the tears and the joy. It is a team effort to get the job done – and to get it done well.

As a myofunctional dentist, my expertise lies around the mouth and face. The mouth and face are part of the head, which sits on the neck. The neck connects the head to the rest of the body. Inside the head, there are many functional structures and systems that are related to the mouth and face, including the airway, the nose, the nervous system, the start of the digestive system, and even the brain.

Am I an expert on the brain? No, I am not – but that does not mean that I am going to ignore its relevance. There are practitioners out there who are experts in brain function. So, why not collaborate and integrate the management plan with them to ensure that the patient receives comprehensive care, especially in children, where all the functional systems are still developing and consolidating? The brain has completed 90% of its growth by age five.

When I first met Ethan, I already had in mind the practitioners I would need to 'recruit' to build a team around him. There were many layers of Ethan that we all had to peel off. These members of the team did not all have to be involved at the same time. They would be needed at different stages of his growth. Nevertheless, I knew that every member of the team would have the same mindset of figuring out which one came first, the chicken or the egg.

It was still early days, and we had only scratched the surface of this story.

CHAPTER 2 KEY FINDINGS

- Every issue in a child's development is connected to others, even when the link isn't obvious at first.
- Finding the root cause often means peeling back several layers and looking beyond the surface.
- Supporting your child's overall wellbeing usually takes a team – different professionals working together to give truly comprehensive care.

3

Looking beneath the surface

How the mouth tells a story

I found out during his initial consultation that Ethan was neurodivergent. He was on the spectrum. This is a neurodevelopmental condition that affects social interactions and behaviors. It is a disorder that begins in early childhood, with signs usually appearing in the first year of life. As these children grow, they may have problems functioning in society.

This explained why Ethan could not look me in the eye. He did not answer my questions and was awkward in his body language. He was not shy; he was only trying to protect himself from the unknown. There was a significant lack of communication skills, and so Sally did the talking. He sat there quietly, but would follow instructions accurately from his mother.

As his mother and I carried on with our conversation, I was subtly observing Ethan. I was using my myofunctional eye and taking mental notes. To me, this part of the initial meeting is one of the most important because the patient is usually at their most natural state, in which they show the ways they use their mouth and face normally, without realizing that they are being watched.

Ethan was looking at the walls, up at the ceiling, and around all corners of the room, making sure that he would not accidentally make eye contact with me. His mouth remained open the entire time, unable to close his lips for even just a couple of seconds. His breathing was heavy and audible, with his head posturing forward and the back of his neck appearing clearly strained. He was using his chest to breathe, taking deep breaths as if he was struggling for air. When he swallowed, his tongue was thrusting forward between his upper and lower front teeth, and both his cheeks would push inward to help push his saliva back into his throat. These were all obvious signs of orofacial dysfunctions.

Breathe right, grow right

Orofacial means the mouth and face. When the muscles of the mouth and face are functioning optimally, the tongue postures up against the palate at rest; the lips are closed in a relaxed manner (without straining); breathing is through the nose, quiet, and using the diaphragm; and there are no other muscles needing to work except for the tongue during swallowing.

Healthy functional breathing also leads to better body posture. When Ethan was posturing his head and neck forward, he was trying to widen his upper airway to be able to breathe. He was using his chest to pump the air in and out instead of using his diaphragm. His diaphragm was likely locked, unable to mobilize. Consequently, his breathing was loud and audible, sounding like he needed to put in a huge effort just to be able to breathe. In other words, he was over-breathing.

These dysfunctions that Ethan had were likely also related to the state of his nervous system. His body was under stress, and so his nervous system was dysregulated – he was functioning in constant fight or flight. His sympathetic nervous system was in overdrive.

You have probably heard the phrase 'I peed my pants' when someone got startled. When in fight or flight, the body often responds excessively when frightened. Sometimes the response saves and protects you, and at other times the response is prolonged and beyond the person's control, activating certain organs unexpectedly, such as the bladder. This is when it becomes abnormal. The fight or flight should only be activated when required, not be persistently on.

Sally told me, 'Well, Ethan was wetting his bed nightly until a few months ago. He was still wearing night nappies to sleep back then.' When his mother told me this, I knew he was in a constant state of sympathetic imbalance. He was over-breathing and so not oxygenating his organs sufficiently, and the smooth muscles of his body would go into spasm as a result. The bladder is made up of smooth muscles, resulting in the bedwetting during sleep.

Normal does not always mean optimal

My myofunctional eye kept watching Ethan. There are many layers of dysfunction to look through and beyond. Each apparent dysfunction is likely to be a compensation for another. His tongue was sitting low and unable to elevate during swallowing. Consequently, it was thrusting forward, with the cheeks getting overactivated to perform the swallow mechanism instead. The overactivated cheeks might be the most obvious dysfunction, but in Ethan's case, this was actually a compensation for the tongue thrust, which in itself was a compensation for the inability of the tongue to elevate to perform the swallowing in the first place.

The body finds ways to cope when something isn't working quite right. One problem often hides another, and what we see on the surface is usually just part of the story. Children, especially, are clever at adapting - their bodies learn to compensate so they can keep growing and functioning as best they can. But those same adaptations can make it harder to see what's really going on underneath. That's why it can take time and patience to uncover the true cause and gently help the body return to balance.

With Ethan, he was still functioning and continuing to live a life that was normal to him. Normal does not mean optimal, though. His normal and my normal would be totally different. Everyone has their own normal. It is the state of functions that their body is used to. Every individual's normal functions and postures may not be the ones that they're ideally supposed to have.

The amount of information I had gathered so far was still insufficient. Making the observations of Ethan's orofacial dysfunctions was merely detecting the signs. I needed to get past his normal. I needed to go deeper to get closer to the root causes. He was hiding something obscure, and I had not found it yet.

I was determined to investigate further.

CHAPTER 3 KEY FINDINGS

- When something in your child's body isn't working quite right, it often finds clever ways to compensate so it can keep functioning.
- It can take a trained eye to notice how the mouth, face, and breathing are working together – and where things might be out of balance.
- What seems 'normal' for your child may not always be the most healthy or efficient way for their body to function.

4

Looking back to move forward

I was hungry for more information about Ethan's journey so far. With a playful tone, I warned Ethan that I was going to ask his mother about him and invited him to join our conversation: 'I need to ask your mother about you, Ethan. I will take her back to the very beginning, and if you know the answer to any of the questions, jump in at any time.'

Unsurprisingly, he did not acknowledge me. He sat still, staring blankly at the wall in front of him, as if he was not paying attention. I knew that he was and that he was listening, and understood me.

In my opinion, it is important to ask for permission as much as possible, from the parents, and also from the patient, before asking these questions about their history. After all, we are going to talk about them, in front of them. This not only warns them, but also demonstrates that 'I respect you as my patient'.

As a practitioner, I feel humbled and privileged whenever a new patient comes to see me. Why did they choose to see me in the first place? There are many practitioners out there that can do what I do, but they have decided I am the one who can help them.

Early feeding foundations

'I only breastfed Ethan for three months. He had a weak suck,' Sally recounted. This had been challenging for Sally, and so she switched to feeding him with a bottle instead.

'Did you get anyone to help you with the breastfeeding?' I asked.

'No. I did not know where to get help. I did not realize there would be people out there who could help with breastfeeding,' she replied. Unfortunately, Sally could not find the guidance she needed to improve the breastfeeding experience. She was not even aware of such help being available.

Ethan still needed feeding to keep growing. Babies need this to survive. And so, if one way was not an option, it was logical to choose an alternative. 'I think my supply was low. So, I fed him formula with a bottle. He was doing much better with the bottle, and so I stuck with that,' she recalled.

The World Health Organization recommends exclusive breastfeeding for the first six months of the life of an infant. After that age, the introduction of complementary foods is advised, alongside continuing breastfeeding until at least two years of age.

Breastfeeding should be a wonderful experience for the mother and the baby, and for the whole family. It should not be stressful, painful, or challenging. It is a time for bonding and embracing the love between a mother and her child.

When breastfeeding, the lips need to latch and form a strong seal around the nipple. They should not slip off frequently. The tongue suctions, compressing the nipple and areola to express the milk, drawing it into the infant's mouth by creating a vacuum. A rhythmic movement of the tongue follows to swallow the milk. There should not be any compensatory movements from other muscles of the mouth and face.

The baby should be positioned more upright instead of lying horizontally. This makes sense to me because when I imagine myself drinking while lying down, I would actually choke and spill everywhere. The more upright position also avoids the nose being blocked by the breast falling onto it, meaning that the baby is able to coordinate their suck, swallow, and breathe reflex action.

All of the above, when functioning optimally, also plays a critical role in the growth and development of the face, the upper airway, and the head. When the tongue is functioning as it should, it widens the jaws, keeps the upper airway patent (open and unobstructed), and prompts the cranial bones to decompress and pump fluids within them to flow effectively. The forces that the tongue exerts onto the palate have a knock-on effect that lengthens the base of the cranium, driving facial growth in a favorable direction, which is forward.

A lactation consultant is like a coach for feeding your baby. They help new parents feel confident with breastfeeding or bottle feeding, whether that means teaching comfortable positions, allowing a baby latch properly, or finding solutions for challenges like low milk supply, pain, or fussiness at the breast. They're there to make feeding more comfortable, successful, and stress-free for both parent and child.

Some lactation consultants are skilled in detecting tethered oral tissues in babies, such as tongue ties, lip ties, and cheek ties.

These restrictive oral ties can affect feeding due to the muscles of the mouth being unable to move as well as they should. (More about them later in the book.)

What snoring tells us

During sleep, Ethan would snore with his mouth open. This was telling me that when he was sleeping, his tongue would fall backward, narrowing his airway. For this reason, if he kept his mouth closed with the tongue falling backward, he would not be able to breathe through his nose. The mouth, therefore, would need to open to breathe.

Sally said, 'He sounds like a truck when he sleeps.' Snoring is basically the sound created by air turbulence. This turbulence comes from the upper airway being narrowed or obstructed. The narrowing or obstructions may originate in any part of the upper and nasal airways.

Inside the nose, there are nasal turbinates, which are bony structures covered by soft tissue. Their purposes are to regulate airflow, warm and moisten the inhaled air, and filter the dust and debris entering the nose. Allergies, infections, and chronic inflammation may cause these turbinates to become enlarged, leading to narrowing or obstruction of the nasal passages.

In the upper airway, there are also masses of tissue called tonsils. These are part of the body's immune and lymphatic systems; they trap pathogens or germs entering through the nose and mouth. There are three types of tonsils: the adenoids (located behind the nose, attached to the back wall of the pharynx), the palatine tonsils (located behind the mouth, which can often be seen when the mouth is wide open), and the lingual tonsils (located behind the tongue, attached to its back surface). Similar to the nasal turbinates, these tonsils can become significantly enlarged due to allergies, infections, and chronic inflammation, which then narrow or obstruct the upper airway.

Another possible point of upper airway obstruction is at the level of the tongue. When the tongue is low in posture and low in tone, it can easily collapse backward, especially when the person is lying on their back. 'Is that why he snores?' Sally asked me, 'Because his tongue is falling back into his throat?'

The muscles of the upper airway themselves may have low tone also. These muscles usually relax naturally during sleep, but if relaxation is excessive, the upper airway may collapse or narrow, affecting breathing and, in turn, the quality of sleep.

In 2021, researchers at the University of Maryland School of Medicine found that children who snored regularly (three or more times per week) were more likely to have thinner grey matter in several regions in the frontal lobes. The thinner cortex in these regions correlated with behavioral disturbances associated with Sleep Disordered Breathing (SDB), which include a lack of focus, learning disabilities, and impulsive behaviors. The snoring condition causes disrupted sleep throughout the night due to interrupted breathing and a reduction in oxygen supply to the brain.

I have always wondered if instead of Sleep Disordered Breathing, it should actually be called Breathing Disordered Sleep ...

Why good sleep matters

Sleep consists of two main parts:

1. the Non-Rapid Eye Movement (NREM) phase
2. the Rapid Eye Movement (REM) phase.

The NREM phase is made up of three stages: N1, N2, and N3. The REM phase is a stage on its own. Good sleep involves passing through these four stages in order, as cycles throughout the night.

Stage 1 (N1) is when you are falling asleep. Stage 2 (N2) is when the body temperature drops, heart rate drops, breathing slows, and the muscles relax. Stage 3 (N3) is the deep sleep stage, or the restorative stage, which is important for recovery and growth. Stage 4 (REM) is fundamental for cognitive functions, including memory, learning, and creativity.

Because muscles relax during sleep, if a person has a narrowing or obstruction of their upper airway, the body may run into difficulties breathing at any stage of sleep. Consequently, the body 'wakes up' to restart breathing, resulting in the person not completing the stage of sleep that they are in and instead returning to the beginning of the cycle. If this continues to happen during sleep, especially night after night, the body is unable to recover, unable to grow, unable to develop its cognitive functions, and the organs are not going to receive sufficient oxygenation due to the breathing dysfunction.

Just as I was suspecting about Ethan's quality of sleep, Sally shared with me, 'His bed is usually messy in the morning. I think he moves around a lot during the night.' She was probably not wrong.

'When the body struggles to breathe properly during sleep, the natural reaction is to move, to wake up and start breathing. It's not like he's fully awake and conscious. His body readjusts so he can breathe better again. This happens numerous times a night as his tongue keeps collapsing backward,' I elaborated.

Imagine if you have a child who has a breathing dysfunction. Their sleep is frequently interrupted throughout the night. No wonder they wake up feeling tired and grumpy, and may have behavioral issues during the day. They are exhausted from not having good-quality sleep, night after night.

You should know about and watch for the signs:

- snoring
- loud teeth grinding
- waking up multiple times during the night
- night terrors
- pausing and gasping for air
- restlessness, moving frequently, or kicking during sleep
- bedwetting, even though toilet-trained
- open-mouth posture
- extending their head and neck back while asleep
- feeling hot and sweating.

These are the most common indicators that parents report to me about their children.

These children are in sympathetic overdrive, or in fight or flight, because they are under stress during sleep. When they are awake during the day, they remain in sympathetic overdrive, making it difficult for their fight-or-flight response to switch off. In other words, their nervous system is dysregulated.

Having a sleep study done can help confirm the presence of a sleep disorder. There are different levels of study that patients can have. At the very least, a level-two sleep study is recommended to provide comprehensive, indicative, and definitive results. The more information it can give you, the better it is for working out the treatment options for the patient.

When bedwetting signals a deeper problem

Ethan needed to wear diapers, or nappies, to sleep until he was over nine years old. His breathing and nervous systems were in dysfunction. Not only was he in sympathetic overdrive, as explained above, but his organs were not receiving adequate oxygen. When the body lacks oxygen, it is a condition called *hypoxia*.

With hypoxia, the body is in a more acidic state. Therefore, the body needs to neutralize this by releasing ions to maintain a balanced pH. One way of doing so is by expelling urine, where the smooth muscles of the bladder go into spasm (triggered by the acidity). In children, they are likely to bed wet. In adults, they may wake up multiple times during the night to visit the bathroom.

There are various possible reasons for bedwetting, of course. One is having retained primitive reflexes. These can interfere with nervous system development, bladder control, and sleep regulation. The Spinal Galant Reflex, in particular, is often linked to bedwetting. When retained, light stimulation along the lower back (like from pajamas, sheets, or even body movement at night) can trigger involuntary bladder release. (I will discuss primitive reflexes further as we delve into Ethan's story.)

The hidden work of the tongue

When younger, Ethan also needed speech therapy. His speech development was slow and delayed. In fact, as you are able to gather by now, his overall communication skills were affected. By the time I met him, he was still hardly verbal. I did not hear his voice at all during that first consultation. There was very little movement from his tongue, which I could see because his mouth was always open, except when he swallowed, when the tongue would make an appearance due to the forward tongue thrusting dysfunction.

This led me to another interesting factor in his history. 'It's very difficult for Ethan to swallow tablets and certain foods, especially fibrous ones, like vegetables and fruits. He cannot tolerate them,' Sally said with a concerned look on her face. In my opinion, because he had limited tongue mobility, his tongue was not able to move the foods around in his mouth for adequate chewing. When foods have not been chewed enough, swallowing them becomes challenging. To make things worse, his tongue could not elevate and move rhythmically to form a proper swallowing motion but was thrusting forward instead.

To understand how this would feel, try swallowing your saliva while keeping your tongue down low in the mouth. Do not let your tongue move up at all, especially as you are about to perform the swallow. Have you tried it? Not easy, right? And now put yourself in Ethan's shoes. Imagine him trying to swallow tablets and fibrous foods while his tongue remained sitting low in his mouth. I think you're getting the picture.

Every child's story is unique

Ethan's history was unique to him. Nevertheless, I see many children who have similar histories, where functionally they should be thriving as they grow, but they're not. Finding out the journey that each child has been through is paramount in the process of evaluation and diagnosis. The history forms the foundation of how the treatment options and plan will be formulated for each individual. Everyone has their own unique history, which usually tells us a lot about why and how they have become the person they are now. History alone is insufficient, however, and data needs to be gathered to complete the big picture.

Sally commented, 'I never thought all these things about Ethan were important, especially to a dentist. I can see now why the dentists we have been to just wanted to wait. They just didn't understand how everything is related.' I was pleased to hear her make such a comment. This showed me that it was all making sense to Sally. She appreciated the importance of the journey traveled because it was all unique to Ethan. It was his and his alone.

Do your children have some or all of the signs and symptoms that Ethan had? Maybe they have different ones? Start by recalling their journeys from the very beginning. Yes, even since the pregnancy. Are there any issues standing out to you? Write them down as you go along, because every little event may actually hold a crucial piece of information that tells a deeper tale.

CHAPTER 4 KEY FINDINGS

- Optimal breastfeeding, sleep, and breathing increase the likelihood of optimal functional growth and development.
- An initial evaluation is always required for each individual patient.
- Understanding your child's full history – from feeding and sleeping to behavior and habits – helps uncover the root causes behind any ongoing issues.

5

Understanding the whole child

Collecting the clues

To dot the I's and cross the T's, I needed to gather harder evidence. Just like with every patient, after the initial evaluation, I explained to Sally that more information is required to determine the root causes, the goals, and the options to achieve them. 'There is more than meets the eye. I need to investigate what we cannot see. There is always a possibility of an unexpected finding, which may throw a curveball into our entire game plan,' I explained to her.

In my practice, records mean a set of data, which I can analyze to formulate a plan for each patient. These records are comprehensive, consisting of photos of the patient's bite (from the front and both sides), the dental arches (upper and lower), the tongue (at different elevations and extensions), the lips, the face (from the front, the back, at both angles and both sides), the smile, the height of the patient, and posture (again from the front, the back, at both angles and both sides). Videos are also taken of the patient talking, swallowing, breathing, and moving the tongue in different directions, for the purpose of assessing their orofacial functions and resting postures.

Sally understood and agreed for Ethan to have records taken.

Technology in healthcare has definitely come a long way. As part of the set of records, three-dimensional study models of the patient's teeth and bite are captured using a digital scanner, creating an instant animated accurate representation of the patient's actual oral cavity. These models allow me to measure the widths and lengths of the dental arches, the shapes of the dental arches, how deep the bite is, how far apart the lower front teeth are from the upper front teeth, how high and symmetrical the palate is, and how the upper and lower teeth relate to one another.

To top it all off, digital X-ray machines are now commonly used in dentistry to 'see' deeper. Over the years, newer machines create lower and lower radiation dosages, making them much safer for patients. In my practices, I have specific machines that have the lowest radiation dosage that can produce the best quality of images, ensuring even further safety for the children that we commonly see. And so to complete the records, X-rays are taken of the head and jaws, from at least three different views. If these views aren't sufficient, the machines are also capable of taking three-dimensional CT (computed tomography) scans that allow the practitioner to investigate further, especially if measuring the upper airway volume is required.

More than data

For his record gathering, Ethan saw one of my oral health therapists, a dental provider who looks after the dental health of children and the gum health of patients of all ages. Because we do not do general dentistry, the oral health therapists at my practice take on the roles of orofacial myofunctional therapists, who are health professionals that look after the functional health of the muscles of the mouth and face. They are experts in evaluating the functions and postures of these muscles, and are the personal trainers to the patients who need to undergo retraining of their orofacial muscles.

The retraining program for these muscles is called orofacial myofunctional therapy. It is similar to body training at the gym, but focused on the mouth and face. The patient is assessed at each visit to determine which areas need improvement, then specific exercises are prescribed and demonstrated for the patient to practice. Mouth tools are also provided as needed, acting like gym equipment to help perform the exercises. And yes, each patient has a personal trainer throughout the entire therapy. (More about this later in the book.)

Back to Ethan. So, he did very well throughout the record-gathering appointment. He connected with the orofacial myofunctional therapist and did everything he needed to do with no hassles. Ethan showed a lot of interest in everything that was being collected: the photos, the videos, the digital study models, and the X-rays. The therapist went through them with him, pointing interesting things out to him, like his unerupted future adult teeth that were still growing inside his jaw bones. He was transfixed by the images. Sally became engrossed too, as she listened to this fascinating show-and-tell that the therapist was putting on.

This record-gathering visit acts as a key stepping stone in building the relationship between the patient, the parents, and the orofacial myofunctional therapist. The therapist takes the opportunity to get to know the patient and the parents, providing an environment where they can engage with one another. This strong starting point creates a perfect setup for the eventual treatment to progress favorably and predictably.

Gathering the results

Now that Ethan had his records taken, the therapist assembled all the pieces. 'I am going to sort your images out properly and pass them on to Dr Donny,' the therapist told Ethan. I would then access the file to begin analyzing every single item by tracing them, measuring them, and comparing them to the optimal.

The record analyses took me about 90 minutes to complete. There was a substantial amount of data produced to assist in the diagnostic process. From there, I could formulate a plan with the options available for Ethan and his mother to choose.

Ethan's upper and lower jaws were positioned too far back in relation to his cranium (skull). This means his jaws did not grow and develop naturally forward. Behind the jaws would be his upper airway. Therefore, the size of his upper airway was narrowed, partly because of his jaw positions.

Additionally, his lower jaw was further back than his upper jaw by quite a significant distance. In fact, it was more than one centimeter further back. A sound relationship would have the lower jaw positioned about one to two millimeters behind the upper jaw. Now, the tongue would be attached to the lower jaw, and so it would also be positioned too far backward when the lower jaw was such. The upper airway would then be further compromised by the tongue collapsing back into it.

The widths of Ethan's jaws were also compromised. His upper jaw was extremely narrowed by the excessive inward forces from the muscles of his face, mainly the cheeks. These muscles had been overactivated whenever he was functioning, as they needed to compensate for his tongue.

When the tongue functions and sits low in the mouth and does not push up against the palate (roof of the mouth), the facial muscles need to work harder. This leads to the upper jaw receiving more forces from the outside in, rather than from the inside out.

The lower jaw sits under the upper jaw. If the upper jaw is not growing wide, the lower jaw may become trapped under it or end up wider and/or more forward than the upper jaw. Because the teeth sit in the jaws, their positions and bite are also affected.

You can detect the relationship between the upper and lower jaws by looking at the bite. A trapped lower jaw usually results in a deep overbite (when the lower front teeth are covered by the upper front teeth too much) and/or an increased overjet (when the lower front teeth are too far back horizontally and often cannot even bite onto the upper front teeth at all). A wider lower jaw usually results in a crossbite (when the lower teeth are biting in front of the upper teeth), which can occur on one side of the bite, both sides, or even at the front. When it involves the front teeth, this is commonly known as an underbite.

Ethan had an upper jaw in the shape of the letter V, with a very high and asymmetrical palate. His lower jaw was trapped under it. He had a very deep overbite and an increased overjet. He also had some degree of a crossbite on the right-hand side when his teeth were biting together. His lower and upper teeth were crowded due to insufficient room for them to erupt properly into alignment.

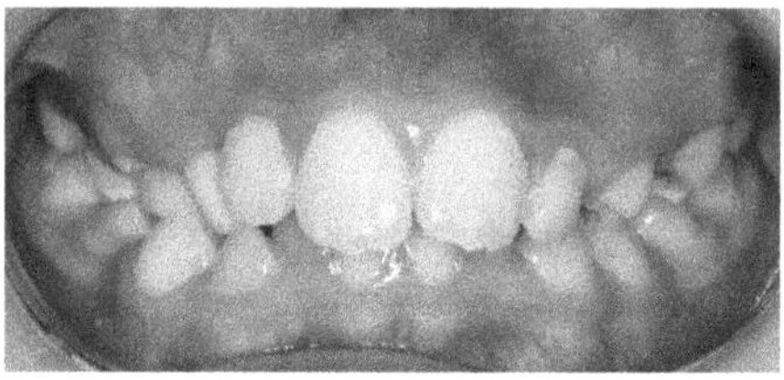

Ethan's bite from the front.

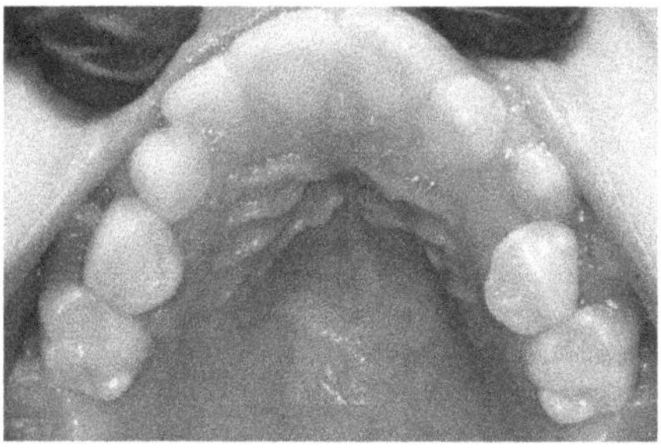

Ethan's V-shaped upper jaw.

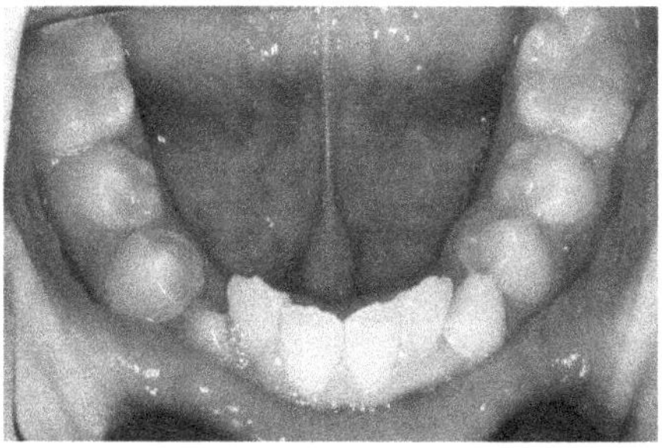

Ethan's trapped lower jaw.

A domino effect

As I mentioned before, Ethan's tongue was a key factor in the growth and development of his jaws. His tongue was also collapsing back into his upper airway because it was sitting and functioning low in his mouth. It also had low tone, meaning that it was lacking the strength to move and hold itself in an elevated position.

The size of his upper airway was, therefore, restricted by his tongue. If he kept his mouth constantly closed to breathe through his nose, he would not be able to inspire (take in) sufficient air. The air entering his nose would move through the inside of his nose, down the back of his nose, continuing down the airway tube to the back of the mouth, before making its way to the rest of the respiratory system. It's at the level of the back of the mouth where the air would face an obstruction from the back of the tongue collapsing into this airway tube. Hence, he kept his mouth open with his lips apart so that he could breathe. It was his body's way of surviving.

Because his body needed more air, Ethan would posture his head and neck forward. The effect of doing this was the opening up of his upper airway further, to ease his already heavy breathing efforts. He was using his chest to pump the air in and out. His breathing was loud and noisy. In short, he had dysfunctional breathing, where his body and orofacial muscles had to work harder to compensate.

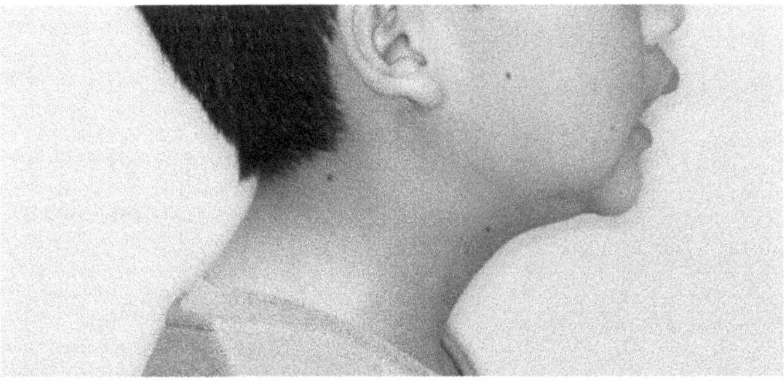

Ethan's forward head and neck posture, and open mouth breathing, at rest.

While I was joining all the pieces of the puzzle together, it became quite clear that there must be reasons for all the dysfunctional patterns Ethan was demonstrating. Yes, there was an apparent neurological issue related to his medical history. And yes, there must be some genetic influence on his growth and development. Likely, epigenetics (more on this later) also played a role.

There was another root cause, though, that was a lot more obvious and actually visible upon closer inspection: a congenital condition that could easily remain undiagnosed by the untrained professional. Not because they missed it, but because they never had the education and training on how to evaluate it.

You only know what you know ...

CHAPTER 5 KEY FINDINGS

- Collecting detailed records helps build a full picture of how your child's structural and functional developments affect each other.
- The record-gathering process isn't just about data – it helps your child feel comfortable, confident, and involved in their own care.
- The way a child holds their mouth and tongue, how their jaws grow, and how they breathe are all closely connected and influence one another.

6

Tied in silence

Are you able to rest your tongue all the way up against the roof of your mouth? Not just the tip of it, but the entire top surface of the tongue actually touching the palate, with a gentle, effortless suction?

Are you able to stick your tongue out and move it side to side without the jaw moving with it? When your tongue sticks out, is there a dimple or an indentation on its top surface?

Are you able to open your mouth as wide as you can and touch the tip of your tongue to the palate without closing your mouth much? Does under your tongue feel tight and sore when you do this?

Ethan was unable to do any of the above easily.

What is a tongue tie?

The tongue is an important organ. When a fetus is forming inside the womb, the tongue is the second muscle to form, after the heart. Its range of mobility, tone, and posture can affect a number of functions, including feeding, breathing, chewing, swallowing, speaking, jaw development, facial growth, cranial movement, and postural fitness.

Under the tongue, there is a band of tissue called a frenulum or frenum. The name comes from the Spanish word 'frena', which means 'to brake' or 'to slow down'. The tongue frenum forms when the fetus is 12 weeks old. In 4% to 11% of the population, the tongue frenum is restrictive to the mobility of the tongue, affecting the organ's ability to rest and function optimally, especially to elevate. When this band of tissue tethers the tongue to the floor of the mouth, it is a medical condition called ankyloglossia, or more commonly known as a tongue tie.

There are other areas in the mouth that can also be tethered. These are the lips and cheeks, as they have attachments too. Just like the tongue, lip ties and cheek ties (also called buccal ties) restrict the movements of the lips and cheeks, respectively, which may cause functional issues as well.[2]

When feeding affects the whole family

When our oldest was born, I had no idea about breastfeeding. I was sitting in a quiet maternity ward, with my wife clutching our newborn to her chest. Her cries had softened after a long, fumbling attempt at nursing. The midwife told us that breastfeeding was

2 I have come across many people not really knowing how to pronounce the word 'buccal' correctly. Buccal means relating to the cheeks. It is not pronounced 'bew-kle.' Simply pronounce it as 'buckle'.

meant to be difficult to start with. 'You'll get the hang of it eventually,' she told us.

We relied heavily on the midwives and the maternal health nurses to teach us about breastfeeding. They kept changing the feeding techniques, the feeding positions, and even got my wife to hire a breast pump to express her breastmilk in the hope she would avoid having mastitis. Top-ups with a bottle would be needed every now and then.

Our oldest did not just feed frequently – her feeds were short, and she would wake up every 40 minutes during the night. At one stage, the idea of attending a sleep school was flagged to us. Oh, and also the suggestion to allow our daughter to cry herself to sleep. 'Stick to a schedule, and don't go and pick her up whenever she cries! Babies are meant to cry, and they need to learn that no one will come to their rescue when they do so too frequently,' one maternal health nurse told us.

I kept thinking to myself that babies wouldn't be able to speak yet, and so crying would be a form of communication. They cry not only because they are in pain, but maybe they are in discomfort, maybe they are in distress, maybe they want something, maybe they are just trying to get your attention, or ... maybe they are hungry ...

Was it the right thing to do to leave our daughter to cry to sleep? Was she actually in so much distress? And if she was, would leaving her alone, not attending to her, make her feel abandoned? Would she then grow up carrying the trauma instilled since she was a newborn?

My wife and I did not enroll in a sleep school. We did not ignore our daughter and let her cry to sleep in distress. Yes, it was tough, and it was taking a toll on our lives. We were lucky that my wife did not have to work. She was dedicated to being with our daughter 24/7. The struggles were all real, and yet we persisted.

Feeding your baby is not just about how the milk gets into his or her body. It's about connection, responsiveness, and love. Many families come to see me because they feel all hope is gone. Troubles affect not just the mother, but often the father as well.

I remember one particular family who came after a long journey without finding answers. The father was visibly suffering as he was so heartbroken, watching his wife unable to feed their baby. He put on a brave front to provide the strength that his wife needed. He sat there not saying many words throughout the initial consultation. He was holding the baby tightly, with so much love flowing deep from his body, as his wife shared their story of trials and tribulations.

My lactation consultant and I were able to diagnose the problem. Yes, the baby had a tongue tie. The latch, the suck, the swallow – all were affected and uncoordinated. We managed the issue definitively and were determined to help as much as we possibly could. We were only a small part of their journey, but we still played a role in changing their path toward the right direction.

With their consent, we released the tongue tie. We then brought the baby back to the family to feed. When the father saw that the mother could breastfeed their baby with no pain, no discomfort, and in fact was relaxed and enjoyed the experience instead, he looked at me and broke down in tears. It was the first time he witnessed his wife breastfeeding their baby without pain. Sure, it was only the first step toward the betterment of their quality of life, and there was still more work to be done. But he hugged me so tight. His tears were flowing down his cheeks, soaking the right shoulder of my scrub top. He was sobbing uncontrollably. 'Thank you ... thank you ... thank you ... ' he kept repeating.

If I could sit with you, struggling parents, right now, across a quiet kitchen table, I would tell you this: 'You are doing an incredible job, even when it doesn't feel like it. You are your baby's greatest advocate, even when your voice shakes. And whatever you choose, it is okay. Because the goal isn't perfection. The goal is love. Nourishment. Connection. A baby held in arms, and a parent who knows they are not broken.'

When my daughter was six months old, a maternal health nurse detected her tongue tie. I had no knowledge of what it was back then. Her suggestion was to have it snipped and see if breastfeeding would improve. So, we did. It was a very quick snip by the nurse, using only her long fingernail. There was no bleeding, it appeared so easy to do, and it was over in less than a second, so that my daughter didn't even have time to realize what was happening. *Wow*, I thought to myself. *It took longer to find a car park than the snipping procedure itself.* I could not believe that this simple stroke would improve breastfeeding and wished that this had been done much earlier.

Well, guess what? It did not change her breastfeeding at all ...

Why tongue posture matters

Yes, Ethan had a tongue tie. His tongue frenum was tight, especially when I felt it with my gloved fingers. He could not lift his tongue up and was resting it low in his mouth. When functioning, his tongue would thrust forward, contributing to the increased overjet that he had.

His tongue never touched the roof of his mouth. He had a weak suck when he was being breastfed for only the first three months from birth. He needed speech therapy. His upper jaw became narrow. His teeth did not have room to erupt properly. His bite was misaligned. He needed to mouth breathe. He postured his head and neck forward to get more air. He was snoring during sleep, as his tongue would collapse back and narrow his upper airway. His sleep was poor, and his bladder remained active while he was asleep.

The ability for the tongue to connect to the palate also has neurological implications, especially regarding how it affects nervous system regulation and even cognitive and emotional states. When the tongue rests against the palate, it stimulates the cranial nerves, in particular the trigeminal and the facial nerves. These nerves feed into the brainstem, influencing the parasympathetic tone. The parasympathetic is your rest-and-digest system, which helps you regulate your stress levels, heart rate, digestion, and even your sleep quality.

When the tongue rests against the palate, it also mobilizes the cranial system like a pump, allowing the fluid around your brain (the cerebrospinal fluid) to flow. This fluid flow also activates the brain's waste system, called the glymphatics, draining waste products into the lymphatic system, especially during sleep. As a consequence, it promotes recovery and healing of the brain.

The tongue connects to the hyoid bone, which is linked to cervical spine positioning. In a male, the hyoid bone is more pronounced compared to in a female. It is commonly known as the Adam's apple. Improper tongue posture can subtly affect body posture, balance, and neuromuscular feedback to the brain.

In a growing individual, the mobilization of the cranial bones also stimulates the cranial base to lengthen, which plays a role in the forward growth of the face. This forward growth also means the upper airway widens, for optimal breathing functions. Therefore, the tongue not only widens the jaws but also contributes to the jaws developing forward.

What seems like a simple resting posture is actually a neurological switchboard connected to deep autonomic and cranial functions.

The question is then: what do we do now?

CHAPTER 6 KEY FINDINGS

- Every tongue has an attachment under it, called a frenulum or frenum.
- Up to 1 in every 10 people has a tongue attachment that is restricting the tongue's functions and postures, called a tongue tie.
- The tongue plays a role in functions and growth since before birth.

7

Cutting ties isn't always the answer

Not all tongue ties need to be released

So, do we end our relationship right here, right now? Have you had enough of being tied down, as if your freedom has been taken away from you? Do you feel like you cannot move, you cannot shine, you cannot lift yourself up and push others to excel? Are you ready to just cut loose and be set free? Or do you need time to prepare before you can show the world who you are, what you are made of, and what you can do?

I am not asking you, the readers, these questions. I am asking the tongue that has a tongue tie. A tongue that is tethered and unable to move with its maximum potential. A tongue that sits low in the mouth, straining to elevate. A tongue that cannot work in the way it's supposed to, making other muscles around the mouth and face work harder.

Yes, having a tongue tie warrants the consideration of having it released. However, the decision to perform the procedure must be determined by how much it has been affecting the functions and the intentions that the patient (and the family) has. Not all tongue ties need to be released.

A few years ago, there was a 15-year-old boy who came to see me because his parents could see a very obvious tongue tie. It was attached to the tip of his tongue. Upon gathering his functional history, however, I found that he had no issues whatsoever. He breastfed with no challenges, he ate with no issues, he spoke clearly without ever needing therapy, his sleeping and breathing were optimal, he had wide jaws and a perfect bite with no dental crowding, no one ever noticed that he had a tongue tie, and he did not have any postural complaints. So, I asked him and his parents if they would like the tongue tie released, considering he was not experiencing any problems from it. They just thought that it would need to be released because they could see it. They actually did not have any concerns about how it looked, especially since not even his family and friends ever realized that he had one. My suggestion was to do nothing.

When I evaluate a tongue tie, I do not make my assessment based on how it looks. How it feels, the range of the tongue's mobility, how it has been affecting the patient functionally or socially, and the patient's and/or parents' desires are all determining factors for whether it should be released or not.

Seeing below the surface

The tongue tie that Ethan had did not look tight or short. It felt tight, though, when I palpated it. When he extended his tongue out, a dimple appeared on the top surface of the tongue, indicating that the mid-body of his tongue was being pulled down by something tight from the undersurface.

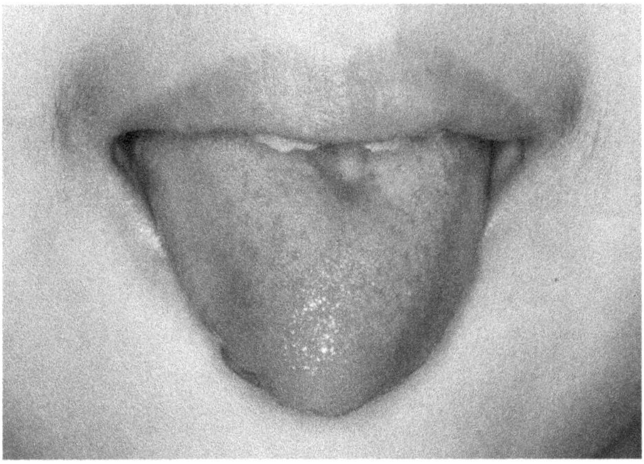

The dimple on the top surface of Ethan's tongue when he extended it out.

His tongue tie was not attached to the tip of his tongue. It was attached about halfway down between the tip and the floor of the mouth. From the front, it looked like a piece of string. But from the side, it looked more like the sail of a boat.

As a matter of fact, every tongue tie is like the sail of a boat. It extends deeper than what can be seen from the front. It is made up of connective tissue, called fascia, which can be considered the inner skin of the body.

The fascia tissue that forms the tongue tie extends between the two strands of the genioglossus muscles, deep under the tongue. This means that when releasing a tongue tie, it is paramount to reach the deeper parts of the tissue to achieve a complete release. Only releasing the part that can be seen from the outside is most likely incomplete.

Everything in the body is linked

Fascia is a complex matrix of connective tissue throughout the inside of our bodies, beneath our skin. It intertwines like tangled cobwebs, lining the surfaces of our internal organs, bones, nerves, blood vessels, and muscles. These fascial layers provide structural support and protection to the body, and are innervated by nerves.

They facilitate movement, allowing muscles to glide under them, acting like shock absorbers and reducing friction between tissues. They are the framework for muscle functions and force transmissions.

There are several fascial lines running through the body. The one that involves the tongue is the Deep Frontal Line. This is the innermost fascial line that runs from the arches of your feet all the way up to the tongue and the base of your skull, covering the diaphragm and the lungs. It serves as the central pole that supports the body, playing a major role in core stability, breathing, posture, and coordination.

At any part of the body, the fascia can become tight, scarred, or inflamed, restricting the movement of not only the part involved but potentially along the related line and possibly beyond. This is because these fascial layers are intertwined, as I mentioned before. Hence, a restriction in one area can usually be associated with restrictions in other areas.

I saw a 44-year-old patient once who had a tongue tie and was determined to have it sorted once and for all. She had many issues that she believed to be related to the tongue tie. One of them was that her knees kept dislocating whenever she would lie down in a supine position. My team and I looked after her with intensive exercises of her mouth and face for a few weeks before and for a few weeks after the tongue tie release procedure. She was also being cared for by her bodyworker, managing her myofascial tensions down her body. After completing her entire program, she was surprised to find that her knees stopped giving way whenever she was lying down. She came back three years later as she wanted to make sure that her muscles of the mouth and face were still functioning and posturing well. 'My knees have not played up since the tongue tie was released,' she reported. This is one great example of how the entire body is a connected system.

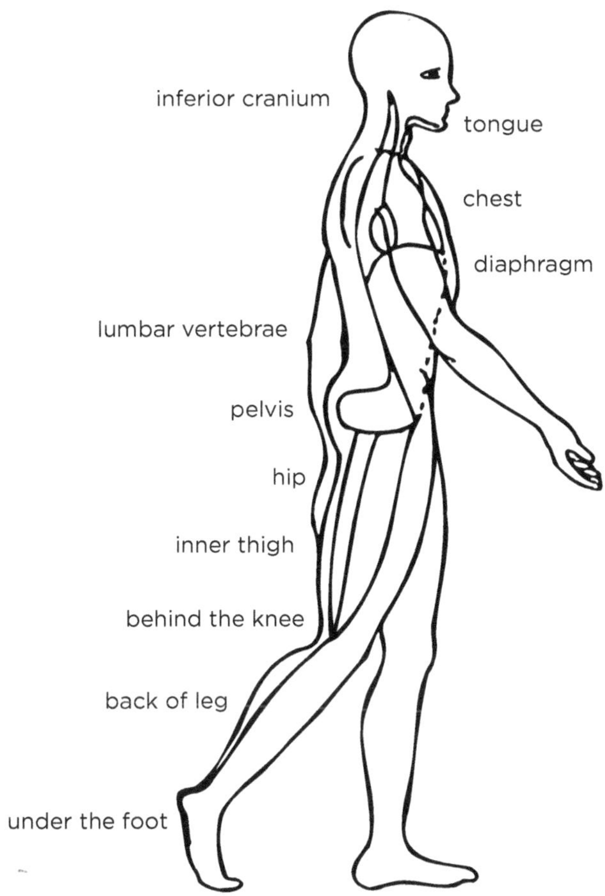

The Deep Frontal Line of fascia.

The power of a care team

Because of this interconnectedness, whenever my team and I are managing a tongue tie, we work closely with a skilled and knowledgeable bodyworker. The bodyworkers we collaborate with are mainly osteopaths and chiropractors who have had extensive training in tethered oral tissues. They assess and treat the myofascial conditions of the patient from head to toe, loosening up tight spots, reducing inflamed areas, and supporting their nervous system. The patient sees them for a few sessions before and a few sessions after the tongue tie release procedure.

As part of the care team, orofacial myofunctional therapists are also involved. They are like personal trainers for the patients, evaluating and prescribing exercises for the muscles and fascial tissues of the mouth and face according to the specific dysfunctions that are present for the patient to practice. This exercise-based approach is known as orofacial myofunctional therapy. These exercises may target the tongue, the cheeks, the lips, the jaw muscles, the facial muscles, the neck muscles, the breathing, the swallowing, the chewing, and often the posture. All of which can help in improving a number of functional health issues, such as poor sleep, snoring, underdeveloped jaws, poor speech, dysfunctional breathing, low tongue posture, low tongue tone, incompetent lips, parafunctional habits, poor posture, and even activating the parasympathetic nervous system (responsible for the body's rest and digest functions) by increasing the vagal tone (the vagus nerve is a key component of the parasympathetic nervous system).

For children under three

In infants and toddlers under three years of age, implementing the orofacial myofunctional therapy is challenging due to their limited ability to comprehend and comply. Between three and five years of age, it can still be problematic depending on the maturity of the individual patient, but it can often be accomplished with the right teamwork and support, especially from the parents.

Hence, for those under three years of age, if the patient requires a release of their tethered oral tissues, it is the parents who need to perform the exercises on their child. These exercises are prescribed to be performed after the release procedure and are crucial in minimizing the risk of the wounds healing back to their original conditions; that is, the ties growing back. Parents are advised to perform the exercises on the relevant areas of the mouth for four weeks, as it generally takes this long for wounds to heal.

The bodywork, as described above, is crucial in minimizing the risk of this occurring. I strongly recommend the bodywork component for patients of any age as part of the oral tie release strategy. I believe their integrative care boosts the chance of achieving more favorable outcomes because of how the fascial tissues are connected throughout the body. As dental practitioners, my team and I are able to treat the head and neck, but we need the bodyworkers to look after the rest of the body.

For children over three

When the patient is over three years old, the orofacial myofunctional therapy is a necessity, in my opinion. Because tongue ties are believed to be formed at 12 weeks in utero (in the womb), the older the patient is, the longer the patient has had the restriction. All the associated muscles have been functioning and posturing suboptimally and in compensation for longer as the patient gets older.

The brain controls the ways muscles move and posture through signals via the nerves. If the brain is used to thinking that the muscles are unable to move and posture in certain ways, it will not send the signals to do so to that particular muscle group. For this reason, when there is a tongue tie that has been anchoring the tongue down to the floor of the mouth, the brain does not normally send neural signals to the tongue muscles for the organ to elevate. And if the tongue tie is released, but the brain still does not send the 'elevation' signal, the tongue remains sitting low in the mouth. Unfortunately, when the tongue remains in this position, the wound from the tongue tie release gets compressed, leading to a higher risk of the tongue tie reattaching.

Having the patient undergo orofacial myofunctional therapy for at least four weeks before the release procedure prehabilitates the brain to establish new neural pathways to the muscles involved. Basically, it gets the brain ready to control the muscles to move in the desired manner once the tie has been released.

After the release, the therapy continues for at least another four weeks to rehabilitate the functions and postures of the affected muscles. This enhances the wound healing as the muscles continue to improve.

Ultimately, the aim of this therapy is to develop automation and habituation of the neural pathways and the myofascial structures. The patient should not need to keep putting in the effort to rest the tongue up against the palate, keep the lips closed, swallow properly, and breathe functionally. These things should become the patient's new normal.

And so with Ethan, I wanted to focus on his root cause as a priority. Despite this, I needed to make sure he would get the best outcome possible because it would determine how the rest of his treatment would progress. His tongue needed to be able to elevate, with optimal strength and tone, increasing the likelihood that it would help in naturally widening his jaws. Not to mention, helping in correcting his associated dysfunctions altogether.

But do we straight away 'cut' the tie? Well, as you now know, that would not be the smartest first step to take.

CHAPTER 7 KEY FINDINGS

- Our inner skin is called the fascia, which covers organs throughout the body.
- The tongue is connected to the toes through the fascia.
- A successful and complete release of a tongue tie requires a program that involves exercises and bodywork.

8

Turning information into action

After gathering and collating all the records, my task was to formulate a plan for Ethan. I spent a bit of time mapping it all out, documenting it, and putting it all down on paper ... well, typing it all up, considering we were not living in the olden days.

Just like every patient going through a similar process, I would provide a treatment proposal that would take every aspect into account. The final product would then be presented to the patient and the parents, verbally and physically, to avoid confusion and ensure clarity.

Understanding the plan for your child's care

In my treatment proposal for Ethan, I outlined his initial presenting concerns. Then his findings were listed one by one, including his history, existing conditions, and measurements, all derived from his evaluation and records. The diagnosis was made, and possible causes were explained. Then his treatment goals were specified, followed by his options.

It is important that patients are always given choices on how to proceed. They do not have to do anything if they do not want to. They are also entitled to seek second and third opinions. As with everybody, my plans are based on and limited to the knowledge and skills I have. This does not mean that there are no better plans available out there, as there may be different approaches that I may not be aware of.

Once the options had been given, I needed to make sure that Sally would be able to make an informed decision. Therefore, I made the treatment recommendation and spelled out what would be involved step by step, from start to finish. The specific associated risks and possible complications would then be discussed, along with an emphasis on the importance of Ethan being compliant throughout the entire treatment period. His parents also needed to know the financial investment they would need to prepare for, and so the fees and payment structure were openly described. All the inclusions and exclusions were itemized clearly.

My treatment proposal used to be about 15 pages long. It was a bit daunting to the patient and the parents, as they would need to spend a while reading through it. Nowadays, it is around seven pages long. No, I did not eliminate sections from it or exclude information. All I did was make the font size smaller. It is now not that daunting.

Understanding the risks and the safeguards

As with any medical and dental treatment, there are associated risks and possible complications. Yes, I already included the specific ones in the individualized treatment proposal. However, there are generic ones that the patient and the parents need to be informed of. Hence, I also provide my patients with a five-page treatment consent document, which comprehensively covers these risks and complications. And you're right ... it used to be eight pages long! You know my trick!

Each human body is unique. When two people undergo the same treatment for the same conditions, it does not mean that they will both respond in the same way. Sometimes complications do occur, although rarely. To me, if the patient and the parents are fully informed beforehand, managing a complication becomes easier.

Understanding what's next for your child

The day arrived when Ethan and Sally came back in for me to present his treatment plan. As I called them in from the waiting lounge, I was feeling excited and nervous at the same time. His plan was extensive, and I was going to recommend the option that would take a long period of time to complete.

I briskly walked out to the waiting room to greet them. Ethan was wearing a thick winter coat. He looked cozy and comfortable with it on. 'How are you both doing?' I gently asked.

'We are doing well. I can't believe how cold it is outside,' Sally replied.

'Lucky the heater is nice and warm in here,' I reassured her. 'Are you ready to go in to have a look at all your photos, X-rays, and scans, Ethan?' I asked, trying to look him in the eye. Ethan did not respond. He sat there quietly until Sally asked him to get off the chair. I led the way down the corridor, and they followed me in.

My room did not have a door; it had curtains instead to separate it from the hallway. They gave a feeling of softness, and patients would comment on how comfortable they made them feel.

I drew the curtains to the sides, opening the path for Ethan and Sally to enter my room. Ethan knew where to sit. He sat in the middle of the room. Sally settled herself in the chair next to him. There was a large monitor in front of them, mounted on the wall. On the screen was a photo of Ethan smiling, the one that the therapist took during the record-gathering appointment. 'Do you recognize who that is, Ethan?' I attempted to break his wall.

Did I succeed? Of course not.

Following a brief, friendly chat with Sally, I began to show them both the records. I explained every finding, every measurement, and every detail, pointing out relevant information to help them understand. From the photos of his posture to the line tracings of his X-rays, I did not miss anything.

Ethan kept quiet throughout the 45-minute appointment, but he appeared to be interested and somehow engaged by everything I shared, especially when we were going through his X-rays and study models. He loved the way I could rotate his animated jaws, teeth, and bite to view them from different angles. At one stage, we were all looking inside his mouth from his throat. The wonder of advanced innovations! He did not mutter a word, and yet he was clearly captivated by all the technology.

Sally was totally engrossed in the discussion. She wanted to know more. She was determined to do all she could for Ethan. Her eyes twinkled with every glimpse of hope. Her body was leaning forward, sitting on the edge of her seat, eager to absorb as much as she could. She asked very little, nodding her head at the end of all my sentences. I could feel her shoulders dropping with relief, her face softening with calmness, and her breathing slowing down with ease. The answers she had been searching for were finally being provided. They all made perfect sense to her, and she could not hide her joy.

I went through every aspect of the plan with them. As I handed Sally the documents, she asked me, 'When can we start?'

Supporting your child through each stage

My plan for Ethan was lengthy. I went through the steps with Sally, while Ethan appeared to be listening as far as I could tell. 'I would like to focus on his tongue tie initially. He is to commence with at least four weeks of intensive exercises of his mouth and face, and begin to see a bodyworker at the same time. The tongue tie release procedure will follow, and another four weeks of rehabilitative intensive mouth and face exercises after that. A removable upper jaw expander will be next, to widen his upper jaw more quickly, considering he is already 10 years of age. I am hoping this mechanical jaw expansion phase will take around six to nine months to complete. Then, I am planning for him to undergo myofunctional preorthodontics, where we will train his tongue to replace the expansion device. In other words, his tongue will be trained to posture and push up against the palate to continue the jaw development naturally.'

By this stage, I started to lose Ethan. Hence, I switched my body position to face him. I became more animated to keep him engaged. My hands were gesturing how wide his jaws would be as I continued, 'The preorthodontic phase will involve you wearing a silicone mouthguard for two hours daily while awake and to sleep every night. You will need to keep exercising the muscles of your mouth and face. We will get you to continue doing so. The mouthguard will act like exercise equipment, encouraging your tongue to lift up and keeping your lips and cheeks away from the jaws. The effect is usually the jaws naturally widening due to appropriate forces being applied to them by these muscles.'

Sally maintained her concentration intensely. Both she and I could sense that Ethan was back in the conversation. Before I lost him again, I proceeded to wind up my explanation: 'Once he is functionally stable, which may take another 12 months, he will then wear the mouthguard to sleep every night to maintain the direction of his jaw growth and functional health. Braces or clear aligners may be needed to eventually straighten and align his adult teeth after he has lost all his deciduous (baby) teeth. If so, he will need to wear retainers for life to prevent relapse of the adult teeth.' Sally leaned further forward in her seat, showing me that she was keen to begin.

Besides the bodyworker, I suspected Ethan would need to see an ear, nose, and throat specialist to have an airway assessment, a breathing educator to specifically correct his dysfunctional breathing, and a speech therapist to assist in developing his speech, at the very least.

The bodyworker I referred Ethan to was a neurodevelopmental pediatric chiropractor. These chiropractors are very niche. They work on the nervous system of children. They are gentle in their treatment and avoid heavy manual adjustments on their patients. They are usually skilled in cranial and fascial release techniques. Their role is to nurture the natural functional and neurological growth and development of children, from newborns onward.

And so, the plan was all set and ready to go. I was prepared to take things slowly with him. I did not want to overwhelm the parents either, even though Sally appeared to be up for anything at that stage. So I decided to only collaborate with the bodyworker to start with, and not refer Ethan to the other practitioners yet.

Before making a decision right there and then, I encouraged Sally to go home and discuss the plan with Ethan's dad. I handed over the plan, all typed up. Yes, all seven pages of it. And I included the consent document in the folder.

I would prefer both parents to understand the entire plan completely and be on the same page before making any decisions. There is nothing worse for the patient than the parents having opposite beliefs, not to mention how confusing it can be for the care team to navigate.

Sure enough, Sally called the very next day to arrange all of Ethan's appointments. She could not wait to help her son thrive while he still had the chance.

But little did we know that nothing was to go according to plan ...

CHAPTER 8 KEY FINDINGS

- Clear goals help you understand what your child needs and what the treatment plan is aiming to achieve.
- Every child is different, so the treatment plan should be tailored to your child's unique needs and situation.
- The decision to move forward is always yours as a parent – made together with your child and in a way that feels right for your family.

9

Time for lift off

No holding back now

It's take-off time for Ethan. His first mission, should he choose to accept it, was to learn how to become aware of his tongue, how it's moving, how it's sitting, and how he is using it. He also needed to understand how he was breathing, and how he was incorrectly using his mouth and chest to breathe.

I assigned a dedicated orofacial myofunctional therapist to become Ethan's personal trainer for his mouth and face. He already knew the therapist, as she had gathered his records for him. She reassessed his dysfunctions and prioritized exercises for his tongue and breathing at his first treatment visit. These initial exercises were simple for him to follow.

The therapist was well prepared. She had met Ethan before and understood communication would be a challenge. Even so, she remained motivated to engage with him, making sure he would feel safe and comfortable with her. Her role was not only as his personal trainer but also as his advocate and ally, whom he could trust. Building this relationship was pivotal in increasing the chance of success.

To accentuate the outcome of the appointments, the therapist also ensured Sally was receiving training. At home, she would be the one laying down the schedule and supervising Ethan whenever he was required to practice the exercises. There were seven exercises he needed to carry out three times daily.

Ethan was also given several tools to use. These were like gym equipment for his mouth. The tools were chosen according to the exercises prescribed. New tools would be introduced as required at subsequent visits.

At the end of the first appointment, Ethan was given written, step-by-step instructions on how to perform the exercises. He also received a chart to complete, ticking a box each time he finished a routine and bringing it back to his next appointment. This helped make him accountable for doing the exercises regularly.

The therapist and I had reiterated on multiple occasions that the therapy was similar to going to the gym. If you joined a gym but never went, nothing would happen. If you went but just watched television at the gym, nothing would happen either.

Peeling back the layers of compensation

'How have you been since I saw you last time, Ethan?' the therapist asked him as he sat down in the chair. Without answering her directly, he looked away but gave a slight head nod, signaling to her that he had been good. He took a deep breath through his mouth, followed by a loud swallow, where his tongue was thrusting forward between his upper and lower front teeth. Sally answered for him, 'He's been great. He's looking forward to seeing you today.'

At the beginning of every therapy visit, the therapist strikes up a conversation with the patient and the parents. Not only does this strengthen the relationship, but the therapist takes this opportunity to assess the patient's orofacial dysfunctions without the patient even realizing it.

You see, these dysfunctions are best evaluated when the patient is in their most natural and normal state. These dysfunctions would not be in their true forms if the patient were asked specifically to do certain functions, as they might 'act' the movements instead.

One dysfunction may also be a compensation for another. For this reason, it is crucial to evaluate them at the start of every visit. When one dysfunction gets corrected, an underlying different one may become apparent. However, it is often difficult to distinguish between a root cause dysfunction and a compensatory one. For example, a patient may present with an open mouth posture, incompetent lip seal, mouth breathing, and a low tongue position. Which one of these is actually the root cause, and which ones are compensating? Perhaps because the tongue is sitting low in the mouth, the back of the tongue is narrowing the pharyngeal airway, causing the mouth to open to allow for better breathing, resulting in mouth breathing and the lips being unable to close competently? Or is it the other way around? At the end of the day, a well-trained therapist with a sharp myofunctional eye makes all the difference. These therapists are skilled at detecting the dysfunctions apparent at that particular point in time and managing them by prescribing appropriate exercises, while keeping an open mind to the possibility of other hidden dysfunctions revealing themselves subsequently.

Building momentum

When Ethan and Sally returned for his second visit one week later, he brought in his completed chart. He was very compliant and demonstrated the exercises well when the therapist asked him to show her. He did everything he needed to do.

'This is wonderful, Ethan,' the therapist commended him. 'You filled your chart in beautifully. I can see that you've been practicing your exercises every day.' Sally interjected, 'I am very proud of him. He would do the exercises whenever I told him to, and he filled the chart in himself.'

The therapist had a good conversation with Sally while observing Ethan functioning as he normally would from the corner of her eye. She then shared with both of them what her findings were and set out the goals for the week: 'Ethan, I can see that your tongue is able to lift up a little more. We still need to work on it and on your lips closing together. We are going to continue working on your breathing, too.' The plan for the visit was being set out by the therapist.

New exercises would then be prescribed and taught, for Ethan to practice three times daily. More exercise tools might be given, depending on the new exercises. He would need to continue filling in his chart and bring it back again to the next appointment.

Each visit, the process would repeat. The goals and exercises would change as his orofacial functions and postures improved. This also meant that the exercises became more challenging from one visit to the next. Of course, compliance would be a determining factor in how Ethan was progressing. Without compliance, progress would be slow or even stall.

Progress photos and videos of the mouth, face, and posture were taken every few visits. The purpose of taking them regularly was not only for record-keeping but also to be able to show the patient and the parents that changes were occurring. It would be difficult to see the changes without comparing the photos over time.

And when they could see the differences, they would be motivated to keep going.

Just to remind you, Ethan had poor levels of communication and social development. My therapist and I were surprised to find that he was very compliant with everything we asked him to do. So, I asked Sally, 'How have you been managing to get him to do the exercises routinely and well?' She said, 'Easy. Every time after he has done them, I tell him that his teeth look straighter. And so, he gets motivated to keep doing them.' Then she whispered to me with a slight grin, 'I actually don't even know and can't even see if his teeth are straighter or not ... '

Forms and functions are inseparable

After four weeks of orofacial myofunctional therapy and being concurrently cared for by the bodyworker, Ethan was ready for his tongue tie release. This procedure is known as a frenectomy. What my team and I do is specifically called a functional frenectomy, because it is not only about the release procedure itself, but it involves the prehabilitative exercises, the rehabilitative exercises, and the bodywork support. When the release is approached from a functional focus, the chance of the patient healing and improving well is increased.

If a practitioner releases a tongue tie on older children and adults without the supportive therapies, they are unlikely to understand functions. In infants, it is impossible to get them to practice the exercises. Hence, with infants (usually under three years old), the bodywork is still necessary, but the parents need to exercise the involved muscles after the release procedure (known as active wound management) to teach the muscles what to do and guide the wound healing. There are some infants who may be slower in improving, and they may require more therapies from appropriate specialists, such as lactation consultants, feeding specialists, or oral motor therapists. Addressing the tie alone means approaching it solely from a structural point of view, failing to recognize the importance of the functions.

Think back to what happened with my oldest daughter from a few chapters back. Her breastfeeding did not improve after her tongue tie was snipped. My wife and I were never told about bodywork, nor about active wound management. We were oblivious to the need for these. But the nurse who performed the release was not aware of them either. So, she did not do anything wrong. She just did not know.

Forms and functions cannot be separated. They should be considered as one at all times. Forms follow functions; functions follow forms.

A common misconception about this notion is the belief that widening the palate fixes breathing dysfunctions. Widening the palate is a structural treatment that makes the spaces larger for the tongue to sit in the mouth and for the air to flow through the nasal passages (the roof of the mouth and the floor of the nose are made up of the same bone). However, widening the palate does not mean the tongue will automatically sit up against it. It also does not mean you will automatically breathe correctly. The tongue and the breathing need to be retrained functionally for these to improve, get corrected, and become habituated.

Having a tongue tie release falls into the same category. The tongue has been anchored down in the mouth since around six months before birth. Releasing the tongue tie alone does not mean the tongue will automatically know how to posture and function correctly. For functions to improve, training is required.

Ethan begins to transform

Before I go any further, I would like to share with you that something interesting began to happen with Ethan. By the fourth weekly visit, my therapist and I noticed that he was making eye contact with us during the appointment. His eyes were glistening with sparks of energy, shining and declaring that he was present right there with us.

Ethan was transforming. His lips were mainly closed together. His breathing was quieter. His head and neck were posturing more upright. He was paying more attention to the people around him. He looked more comfortable in his surroundings. He was walking with more confidence. Something had definitely clicked. His dimmer switch was slowly but surely turning in the right direction. The wires were beginning to fire. I could imagine that his nerve synapses were gradually connecting.

I see this happening over and over again with my patients. The combination of functional therapies from the bodyworker and my team is often enough to turn the patient around – a confirmation that functions can never be isolated from the overall picture.

'Do you know what we are planning to do next week, Ethan?' I asked him about his scheduled tongue tie release procedure. He looked at me and made a slight grin to show his approval.

He was on his way, and nothing could hold Ethan back.

CHAPTER 9 KEY FINDINGS

- Myofunctional therapy starts from where your child is right now and moves forward step by step, setting small goals at each visit to build lasting changes.
- How your child's mouth and face are shaped affects how they function – and the way they function can also influence their development.
- Combining bodywork with myofunctional therapy can support your child's progress on a deeper level, helping both the body and the brain work together more effectively.

10

A closer look at tongue ties

Choosing the right approach for your child

A frenectomy can be performed to release ties in the mouth. In Ethan's case, his tongue needed one. The hope was for his tongue to eventually lift, sealing his mouth and widening his jaws. Not only that, but to help him also achieve optimal functional health.

There are a number of tools that can be used to release a tongue tie. Some prefer scissors. Some prefer blades. Some prefer lasers. Do these tools determine how well a release can be accomplished? Yes ... and no.

It is commonly believed that it is not about the tool, but about the person using it. Any tools can be used to perform the procedure as long as the practitioner is skilled and knowledgeable.

In my opinion, it *is* about the tool, and it *is* about the practitioner. It is also about understanding the anatomy of the tie, how to use the tool, healing physiology, the associated risks, the possible complications, the family dynamics, and, most importantly, understanding the patient.

If the patient or their family are not ready, I would guide them through the necessary steps to prepare or even give them more time to decide.

Anatomy of a tongue tie

When you look at an attachment under the tongue, it appears like a string. The string can be thick, thin, short, or long. It can be attached to the tip of the tongue, one-third of the way down from the tip, halfway down, or even hidden under the base of the tongue.

It is a tie when it restricts the mobility and functionality of the tongue. If it is not restricting these two aspects, it is not a tie; it is an anatomical frenum that we all have.

The pink outer surface of the attachment is part of the layer that covers all the soft tissues in the mouth. This is called the oral mucosa. Viewed from the side of the tongue, the attachment looks like a sail of a boat. It is bordered by the string at the front, under the tongue at the top, and the floor of the mouth on the bottom, like a triangle.

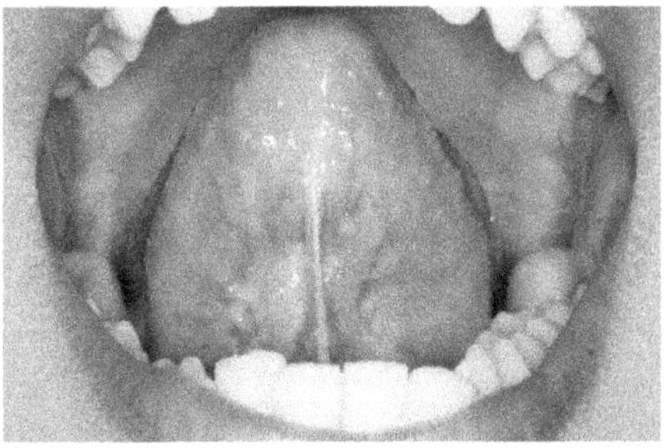

Tongue attachment from the front.

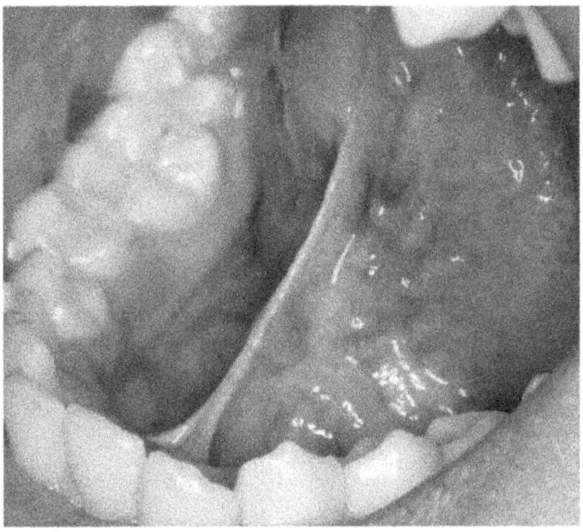

Tongue attachment from the side.

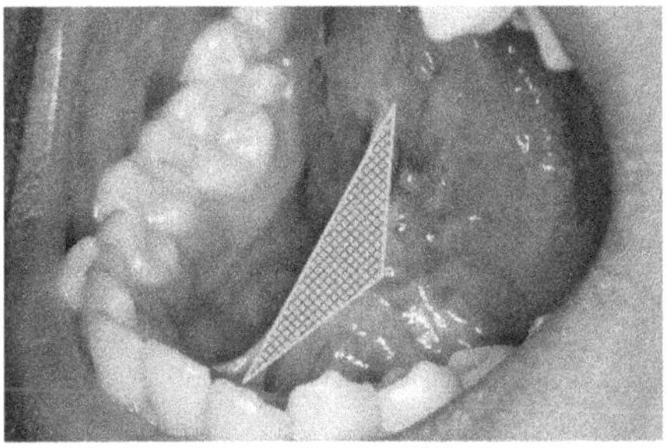

Like the sail of a boat.

Underneath the oral mucosa is the fascia, the connective tissue that is like the inner skin of our body. The fascia is the tissue that can be tight and restrictive, resulting in the tie. It extends deep to cover the genioglossus muscles of the tongue. There are two strands of the genioglossus, one left and one right, with a space in between. Viewed from the front, the strands run vertically, like two pillars under the tongue. The midline space between the two pillars is where the fascia may also continue to extend.

Right in this area under the tongue, there are blood vessels and nerves supplying the structures. Sometimes they may be positioned above the fascia that extends between the two pillars.

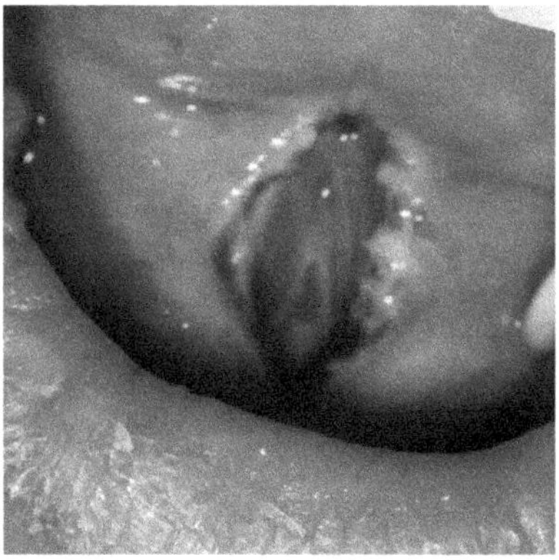

Fascia layers still covering the genioglossus.

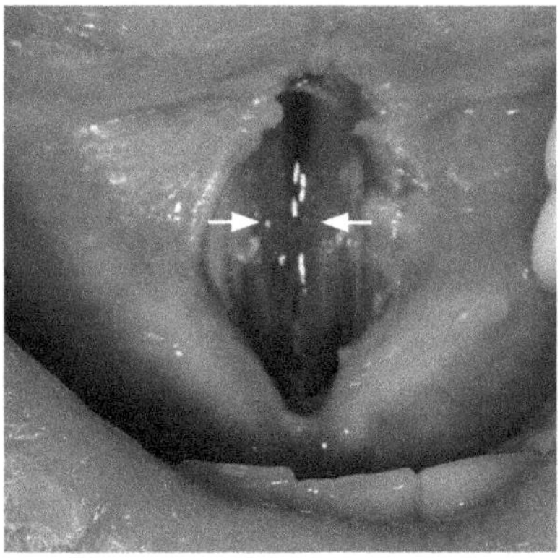

The two pillars of genioglossus with the midline space.

Why a thorough release matters

As you can imagine, when the tight fascia needs to be released, it requires the tool and the skill to reach the deepest tissues safely to achieve a complete release. I can confidently say that I have not yet seen a simple snip with scissors or a blade being able to release the tie fully. This is partly why my daughter didn't see improvements after her tongue tie was snipped.

Using scissors or a blade can release the sail of the boat that is on the surface. When this sail collapses after the snip, it appears as if the tie has been released. However, the deeper fascial tissues are still hidden under the collapsed sail. If the scissors are used to cut deeper from the get-go, there is a risk that underlying structures, such as a blood vessel or a nerve, may be accidentally cut as well, simply because they are not readily visible from the surface.

You can release a tongue tie with scissors or a blade, but it requires time to do so gradually, opening up layer by layer slowly to avoid complications – not just simply snipping it in one second. To perform the procedure properly with such a tool may take around 20 minutes, and the practitioner needs to be highly skilled to navigate through the site. It is a bit like trying to diffuse a ticking bomb ... do you cut the red wire or the blue wire? There is no turning back if you cut the wrong one. The decision may have to be spontaneous and swift while under the pressure of time.

With a laser, it takes around 10 seconds to release a tongue tie, with a lot of pinpoint accuracy. The laser I am using penetrates less than 0.1 mm deep, removing the layers quickly but safely. If a large blood vessel pops up, I can easily take my foot off the pedal to stop the laser instantly. If possible, I can maneuver around the vessel to release as fully as possible.

I have seen posts and videos on social media of tongue ties being released. Unfortunately, it is not uncommon that I come across footage of a tie being incompletely released. If there is still a white layer of tissue covering the muscle bands, the tongue is likely still to be restricted.

Understanding the tools used in a tongue tie release

Lasers work through a process known as ablation. With the laser that I am using, the light gets attracted to water molecules, zapping them off, leading to the tissues separating and loosening. I also prefer to have water gently spraying the site as the laser works. This cools down the area, preventing heating and burning of the tissues, resulting in significantly less thermal damage.

Scissors and blades tend to physically crush the cells of the tissues. They can be more traumatic and usually result in incomplete release of the tie if they are used incorrectly. Yes, they are the tools of choice for some practitioners. There is nothing wrong with this, as long as the practitioners know how to use them well. As mentioned above, having ample time results in a much better release. So, they can work quite well on older children and adults, but how can this be feasible to do on a baby who is awake and in distress?

Should a baby's mouth be numbed?

An infant frenectomy should be performed as quickly and effectively as possible. The patient is usually awake and swaddled tightly onto a special bed to secure them and stop them from moving. No one likes to be swaddled tight and unable to move. An infant does not either, and so they usually begin crying once this happens. They need to be returned to the mother promptly after the procedure so they can feed, especially since they usually are fasting for at least two hours before having the release done. The reason for the fasting is to minimize the risk of them vomiting or having reflux during the treatment, which can be dangerous.

My preference is not to administer any anesthetic for infants. I do not want them to have a numb mouth, as they need to feed immediately after. Post-release feeding is important to settle the baby and control potential bleeding from the wound. One more advantage of having a laser with water cooling is that there is very little discomfort from heat. Plus, the laser actually has a localized numbing effect on the release site.

One of my colleagues actually tried the laser to release her own upper lip tie without an anesthetic. She described it as like pins and needles, with no pain, and her wound felt numb for a couple of hours. There are providers that use lasers without water, and they tend to need to numb the baby's mouth. This helps in reducing the pain, but it can compromise the feeding afterward.

At the beginning of my tongue tie journey, I used to use a laser that did not have water cooling. I still remember to this day that the babies cried very differently because they could feel the heat from the laser. They sounded like they were in a lot of discomfort, adding to an already stressful situation. Their cries were high-pitched. After a couple of infants, I decided to upgrade my laser machine, as I wanted to make the experience as pleasant as I could for these babies and the parents.

The support team

I insist on always having a qualified lactation consultant to co-evaluate and co-manage infants with me. Lactation consultants are the experts in feeding, whereas I am not qualified in the field. Nevertheless, feeding goes hand in hand with oral ties. Thus, the appropriate providers need to be present simultaneously to look after the patient and their parents.

The lactation consultant also assists during the procedure. They hold the swaddled baby gently and monitor their wellbeing throughout. As the practitioner, I focus on the tie. The lactation consultant focuses on the patient's condition, guiding me to continue or to stop depending on how the patient is responding. They bring the baby back to the mother after release for immediate feeding and help to improve the quality of the post-operative feeding experience, along with providing guidance on post-operative care.

My dental assistant is the third person present while the release is being performed. They secure the baby's jaws to prevent them from closing down on the laser, suction the water from the baby's mouth using an oral vacuum, and ensure that my field of vision is adequate to perform the procedure.

The three of us make the ideal clinical team for infant oral ties.

Ethan's big day

Ethan was not a baby, as you know. His tongue tie release procedure was conducted differently from that of an infant. He had had the tongue tie since before birth, meaning that it had been restricting his functions for almost 11 years.

On the day of the procedure, Ethan and Sally arrived earlier than when he was due. He had an adjustment from his bodyworker the day before. They patiently waited until I was ready to see them. As I greeted both of them, I remember Ethan gave me a little smile. His smile said to me that he felt safe and unworried. By that stage, he had been attending our clinic five times, once a week. He knew everyone. The relationship was strengthening.

I brought them into the consultation room first. He sat down in the armchair. It's the most comfortable chair in the room. 'Great choice!' I said to him. I bought the chair from Ikea before I opened the practice. I still have it now, and it is still serving my patients well. It has a high back, where you can sink yourself into it. My patients love it, and some have fallen asleep sitting on it. Sorry I digressed, but it is seriously a great chair if you happened to be in the market for one.

Sally told me that Ethan was looking forward to this. He had been practicing his last set of exercises diligently. I commended him on his efforts, and he nodded to show his appreciation. I could see he was proud of himself, and he was so pleased that I was happy with him.

So, I asked Ethan to demonstrate a few of the exercises he had been practicing, especially the tongue ones. He did them all in the best way possible, considering he still had the tongue tie. I did notice that his tongue elevation was improving already, although not quite there yet. The fact that he could do them well told me that he was actually truly dedicated to his routine. It also indicated that he was ready. The neural pathways to his orofacial muscles were well prepared. These nerves were wiring, primed to fire as soon as the tie was released.

Helping the child feel calm and confident

Most of my patients would be nervous at this point. I would acknowledge their nervousness and let them know that it's only expected because they likely had never had this done before. This acknowledgment usually puts them at ease, as they feel like I truly am on their side and understand their feelings.

I believe it is crucial to explain the process to the patient and the parents step by step. There is no need for any surprises. I would rather the patient understand fully what was happening. The more they know, the more they will comply and be cooperative.

I got Ethan's permission for me to go through these steps. Hence, I proceeded to describe them. 'When I take you into the room, Ethan, I will be taking a few photos of your tongue first. I will also measure how high your tongue can lift up using a ruler. My nurse will be there as well, and she will be helping us out. We will give you a pair of laser goggles to put on to protect your eyes. I will then recline the chair so you can lie down and relax. Then, I will make your tongue tie sleepy by rubbing a cream that tastes like bubble gum. I will be rubbing it on your tongue tie using a cotton bud. Now when you sleep at night, you usually have a pillow to rest your head, right? Well, if your tongue is falling asleep, then we need to give it a pillow to rest. So, I will place a pillow inside your mouth, on the left-hand side. Your teeth will bite down on the pillow, which also helps to keep your mouth open, making sure your jaw joints do not get tired,' I explained.

'Then I am going to massage your tongue using a tongue massager. While your tongue is getting a massage, I am going to put in a bit of sleepy juice, so your tongue will fall into a deep sleep. Hopefully, it will have a nice dream. It will feel weird when your tongue is falling asleep and when it's asleep. It will feel like your tongue has disappeared from your mouth, but remember that your tongue is still there. Once I know that your tongue is in a deep sleep, we are going to use a light called a laser. The laser that I use is invisible to the human eye, so we cannot see it. It's not like in the movies! There will also be water spraying around the laser, and my nurse will have a small vacuum to suck the water from your mouth. You know, actually, your tongue will be having a bit of a pampering. It will be asleep, relaxed, getting a massage, and having a shower! So the shower will be around three to five minutes. I will be starting and stopping during that time as I need to check a few times if your tongue is getting stronger. When the tongue tie is all loose and your tongue can lift up stronger, then I will close the wounds with sutures. This takes another couple of minutes,' I continued.

'While we are doing all of the above, I need you to just close your eyes and focus on your belly breathing, feeling your belly slowly going up and down as you breathe through your nose. When you do this, your body will relax more, and the procedure can finish quickly. At the end, I will take more photos and measure your tongue again. We will then return to this room and show your mum what your new upgraded tongue looks like!' I concluded.

You may have realized that I chose my words carefully. My intention was not to frighten Ethan, nor to make him lose his confidence and courage. At the same time, I would like to let him know exactly the steps, without lying to him. I was being honest with everything I said.

The explanation also made Sally feel safe and that her son was going to be in good hands. The parents would wait in the consultation room and not go into the surgery room with the patient. I suggest this strongly to all my patients. I had allowed a couple of instances where the parents could be present during the procedure. Unfortunately, I had a dad faint when he did not expect that watching his child undergo a medical procedure would make him feel queasy. Suddenly, I had two patients in the room that I had to manage simultaneously! I would rather have just one, please ...

Ethan went in by himself and went through with the procedure without even batting an eyelid. I performed the release in exactly the same steps as the explanation I gave him. There were no complications. He walked out of the room unassisted, unfazed, and with a tongue that could move in ways that it never knew it could.

When we returned to the consultation room, Sally was playing on her phone, looking extremely relaxed and comfortable. Yes, she was sitting in the Ikea armchair. She jumped on the opportunity as soon as Ethan and I walked out of the room, about 20 minutes earlier. I've mentioned already how awesome this chair is. And no, I am not getting paid by Ikea to plug their product.

CHAPTER 10 KEY FINDINGS

- Do not assess an oral tie just by how it looks, but by how it is affecting the functions.
- The practitioner, the tools, and the technique all play important parts in successfully releasing an oral tie.
- A practitioner highly skilled in behavioral management of the patient is likely to be able to perform the procedure with minimal risks and complications.

11

Made to fly

Without the tie anchoring it down to the floor of the mouth, Ethan's tongue took flight. His nervous system was all set to make it fly. The work that he had done with our therapist and the bodyworker had so far been unlocking his unique potential.

Looking after the healing tongue

I went through with Sally and Ethan how to look after the wound: 'The release needed three sutures. It is now healing by primary intention, meaning that it is not an open wound. The sutures will dissolve in one week. However, one or two of them can come loose much earlier because they're under the tongue. The tongue wants to frequently move during functions. You do not have to worry if one or two of them come loose, as the healing would already have begun.

'Now Ethan, you do need to make sure you do not chew or bite your tongue while it is still asleep. And avoid hot foods or drinks. Your tongue will start waking up in about one hour,' I instructed him. Once, one of my younger patients accidentally bit his tongue quite heavily without even realizing it. The wound from the bite was significantly worse than the tongue tie release wound itself.

The wounds take four weeks to heal. Ethan needed to continue with his orofacial exercises to retrain these muscles how to function and posture while the tongue tie wound was healing. In this way, the wound would be guided to heal more favorably, allowing the fascial tissues to repair evenly, providing the necessary gliding mechanism over the underlying muscles for unrestricted mobility.

I pointed out to Ethan and Sally that in the first few days after the procedure, there would be some healing inflammation around the wound, where the edges would look more red and raised. And some degree of contraction of the wound would also be expected as part of the natural physiological process. It would feel annoying because of this every now and then, but especially toward the third and fourth week during the final stages of healing.

The appearance of the wound would also change as the healing process progressed. Within the first week, it would look like a white diamond. The white would then change to a brownish or grayish color in the second week. In the third week, it would change again to a more reddish appearance, followed by returning to the pinkish color of the oral mucosa by the fourth week.

Retraining the muscles for lasting change

'Don't do the mouth and face exercises for the remainder of the day, Ethan,' I added, 'Give these muscles a break today.' The next day, however, he began practicing them again. The same ones that he had been doing for the previous week.

When he came back the week after the procedure to see our therapist, he was prescribed a new set of exercises to focus more on tongue elevation, separating it away from the floor of his mouth. The therapist also began to pay more attention to his cheeks and lips, as these muscles were compensating for the dysfunctional tongue. Therefore, retraining them to correct the compensations would be the logical next step.

As Ethan was able to elevate his tongue further and further, the therapist also worked on his breathing. When the tongue is resting all the way up against the palate, it seals the oral cavity, making it impossible to mouth breathe. Try it yourself: bite your teeth together, touch the tip of your tongue to the gums behind your upper front two teeth, keep this tip there while lifting the middle top surface of your tongue to the palate, then suction the entire top surface of the tongue up against the roof of your mouth, keep the tongue super glued to the palate, then open your mouth slowly without dropping the tongue down, and try to mouth breathe. Are you able to do it? It is difficult to breathe through the mouth when it is sealed by the tongue.

Functional healthy breathing does not only entail nose breathing. It means slow, shallow, gentle, silent breathing, using the diaphragm to pump the air in and out through the nose while keeping the mouth closed and the tongue sealing up on the palate. If any of the above is not happening, the breathing may be dysfunctional.

Keep in mind that breathing and the nervous system go hand in hand. When you are in sympathetic mode, your breathing rate increases, opening the mouth to breathe larger volumes and faster, and often using the chest more to pump the air in and out. This is when you are in fight or flight response. Having this sympathetic response is necessary for certain situations; for instance, if someone jumps in front of you out of the blue and startles you. However, the sympathetic nervous system should not be constantly activated; this means the system is dysregulated and dysfunctional. Sympathetic overdrive is detrimental to your overall functional health.

On the other hand, when you are in parasympathetic mode, which is your rest and digest response, your body is able to regulate, recover, and repair. When your breathing is functional, you're likely to be in parasympathetic, helping you sleep, learn, think, behave, and grow optimally.

Ethan's incredible progress

After Ethan completed three weeks of rehabilitative orofacial exercises, when he came for his fourth visit I thought I had the wrong patient. Standing in front of me was a boy with a wide smile, making consistent eye contact and able to chit-chat with me. I almost shed a tear.

'Great to see you, Ethan,' I greeted him.

'Yes,' he answered.

'I can see your tongue is stronger, your lips are more relaxed, and you are breathing very quietly. I think this is all working out for you, isn't it?' I praised him. He smiled again and nodded his head gently.

Sally did not need to say much. She sat comfortably with a sense of achievement and pride that her boy was blooming. With her own eyes, she was witnessing a transformation that no one expected. Better still, somehow it had only taken eight weeks to get to this point.

His mouth remained closed when he was not talking. His breathing was gentle and quiet. His head and neck were not posturing forward. His cheeks, lips, and chin had noticeably less tension. Remarkably, his jaws were widening and his palate flattening, resulting in his teeth moving toward the right positions. The deep overbite was beginning to open up as his lower jaw was moving forward.

Forms and functions: both or none.

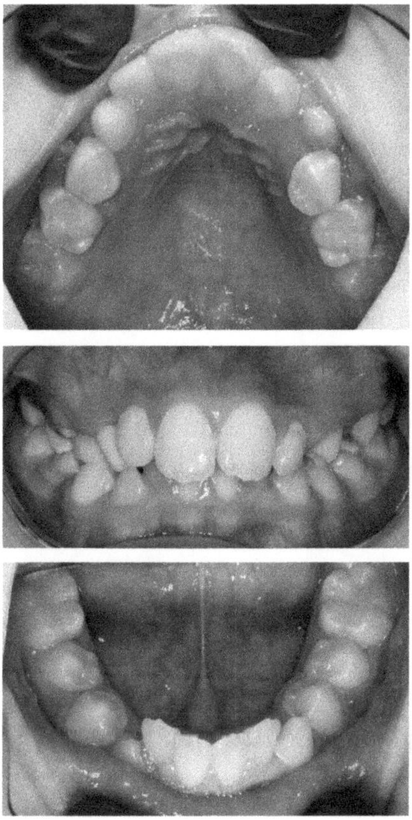

Before commencing treatment.

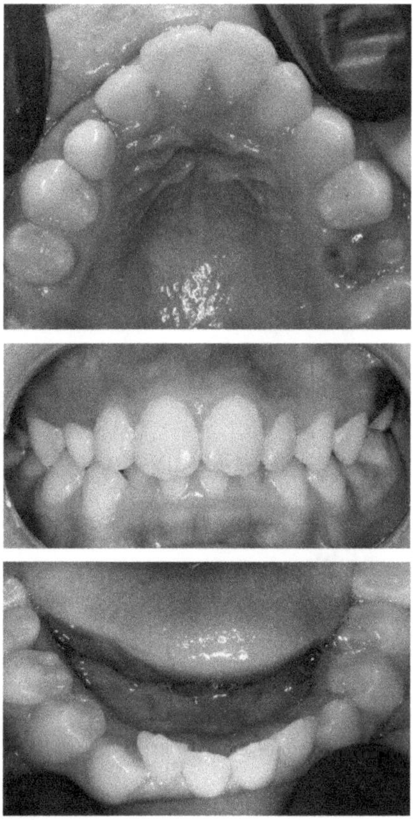

After eight weeks of exercises and tongue tie release.

At that same visit, I was confident his orofacial muscles had improved significantly and would continue to do so. The tone, strength, and mobility of these muscles were close to optimal by that stage. I mapped out my game plan on how to utilize them to boost his jaw development to an even greater extent.

The forces from these muscles needed to be directed appropriately. His tongue would be his best jaw expander. It needed to exert forces up against the palate constantly, shaping his upper jaw to eventually be able to accommodate all of his future adult teeth. The wider upper jaw would also free his trapped lower jaw, allowing it to naturally widen and grow forward.

Originally, as you may be able to recall, I had planned for a removable upper jaw expansion appliance for Ethan to wear after he had completed the initial intensive orofacial myofunctional therapy and tongue tie release phase. How his muscles and jaws were responding by that stage, though, told me I had to reconsider.

I proposed a change in direction to him: ‘How would you feel, Ethan, if I don’t make you an expander yet? I feel that your muscles of the mouth and face are improving so well that I am willing to give them a good go to see if they can work to make your jaws wider instead.’

Ethan replied, ‘Okay.’

Sally gave me a thumbs up.

And so, I got him to start wearing a soft silicone mouthguard. The device had features on it that would attract his tongue to lift up and apply pressure onto his palate, keep his lips forward and away from the jaws, and would push his cheeks out to prevent them from applying forces inward instead.

I instructed him to wear the mouthguard for at least one hour and up to two hours total per day while he was awake. He would need to keep his lips closed over the mouthguard when he was wearing it. This would mean his orofacial muscles would be getting a workout at the same time. For example, he would still need to swallow even with the mouthguard in his mouth, and his tongue would need to elevate to do the swallow due to the device preventing it from moving in any other direction. He would also need to breathe through his nose as his mouth would remain closed to keep the mouthguard in, training his breathing functions simultaneously.

Additionally, because he would be awake while wearing the mouthguard, his muscles would also be trained to keep the device in. This was important because he would also need to wear the mouthguard to sleep every night.

At night, during sleep, growth happens. If the orofacial muscles can exert correct forces on the jaws during sleep, growth is enhanced. The longer the mouthguard stays in the mouth during sleep, the better growth can occur.

And so Ethan needed to begin wearing the mouthguard to sleep as well. He did it on the night that he got the device. Most of my patients would take around eight weeks before the mouthguard would stay in the mouth all night. Well, not Ethan. He kept defying the odds. His stayed in all night, every night, from the first week.

CHAPTER 11 KEY FINDINGS

- Healing takes time – a tongue tie wound will need around four to eight weeks to fully recover after the release.
- Gentle exercises after the procedure help retrain the mouth and face muscles, supporting proper function and reducing the chance of the tongue tie returning.
- As your child's muscles strengthen and work in better balance, they can naturally guide healthy jaw growth and development.

12

Unexpected breakthroughs

Are mechanical jaw expanders necessary?

A jaw expander widens a narrow jaw. Such a device can be removable or fixed (glued onto the teeth). My preference is to use a removable version because it is much better for oral hygiene. Whenever the patient brushes their teeth, the expander can be taken out of the mouth, so the teeth brushing can be done with no interference.

Being removable also means that it allows some degree of movement of the jaw and cranial bones. Fixed expanders are rigid and not flexible, which may result in locking the cranial system up, and overloading the nervous system. I have had patients experiencing headaches and significant discomfort with fixed expanders on.

The downside of a removable expander is that it can be removed easily by the patient, so they may not wear it enough, damage it, or even misplace it. It is very rare for a patient to be like this, but there are a few of them out there. Obviously, if the device is not being worn sufficiently or correctly, the expansion is not going to progress.

It does take time to become comfortable wearing an expander. The tongue tends to play with it for the first few days because it is something new in the mouth. Speech is affected for the first couple of weeks, at least. The mouth hypersalivates initially because it thinks the device is food. After a couple of days of wearing the expander, the mouth realizes that it is not food, and the salivation settles back to normal.

Chewing and eating with the expander in is also recommended. These functions apply forces onto the device, which are transferred onto the jawbone, stimulating it to grow. Using it while eating also means that the expander needs to be cleaned well daily, as food debris gets stuck around its crevices and nooks. I instruct my patients to clean the device whenever they brush their teeth.

Ethan's tongue was low in tone and posture to begin with. His tongue tie was a significant contributing factor. If he were to wear a jaw expander, the device would sit under the roof of his mouth, resulting in his tongue not being able to elevate all the way up against his palate. Not only would this keep his tongue low, it would also break the neurological connection between the tongue and the palate.

I was also mindful of all the work he had done so far. There would be a chance of undoing the tongue retraining to some degree if he were to wear a jaw expander. Ultimately, my aim was to establish his tongue elevation against his palate. Because his progress was very promising, why should I not continue down the current path instead?

To me, wearing a jaw expander is like playing catch up. If the jaw is severely narrow, the expander mechanically forces it to widen more quickly. I do not use these expanders on all patients. In fact, I only use them about 25% of the time, mainly if the patient is older, has minimal natural growth potential, or has significantly inadequate room for the tongue to sit up against the palate. Oh, and when the patient is not compliant with the exercise-based treatment.

The tongue is still the best expander of the jaw. And it is actually already built-in inside the mouth. It just needs to be trained to apply forces to the right places for it to expand the jaw. So, the tongue is the natural version, and expansion devices are the mechanical version of jaw expanders.

Training muscles, not just making space

Many parents have brought their children to see me for jaw expansions. The common belief is that expanding the jaw alone can treat the breathing and sleeping issues. Hence, many think that expanding the jaw is the cure for the functional problems their children are facing.

Expanding the jaw using mechanical devices can definitely make the jaw wider. However, it does not correct the functions. Creating the space for the tongue to fit is wonderful, but does it know how to position and work itself properly?

Without training the tongue, if it has been sitting low in the mouth for a long time, it does not automatically know how to elevate, even when it has been given the room to do so. The signals being sent to the tongue have been controlling it to stay down. These signals need to be rewired to control the tongue and make it elevate instead.

The same goes for the other orofacial muscles, especially those that have been in a compensatory state. For example, when the tongue sits low, unable to elevate to swallow, the cheeks and chin may need to work harder during swallowing to compensate for the tongue. Thus, training the cheeks and chin becomes necessary to eventually eliminate the compensations, which helps in elevating the tongue further. Everything is connected and works in unison to achieve the goals.

When Ethan underwent the intensive orofacial myofunctional therapy over eight weeks (four weeks before and four weeks after the tongue tie release procedure), the exercises targeted all of his possible dysfunctions simultaneously and gradually. It would be insufficient to only exercise one muscle per visit. Treating only one dysfunction at a time would hinder the progress of the therapy because associated dysfunctions and compensations would be ignored.

A whole-body approach

In my early days, when I began learning about myofunctional dentistry, I was taught to only teach the patient one exercise per visit and see them once a month. The exercises were also very rigid in sequencing and goals. The first three monthly visits would focus on the tongue, prescribing one tongue exercise per visit. The second three monthly visits would focus on the lips. The next three monthly visits would focus on breathing. Then the final three monthly visits would focus on posture. Every patient was expected to complete the treatment in exactly 12 months. And all of them were expected to do the same exercises in the same order.

As you may have figured out, that system was heavily flawed. It failed to recognize the presence and interconnectedness of multiple dysfunctions and compensations. Moreover, it failed to understand that not all patients have the same dysfunctions. Because of this, my success rate was extremely low. Hardly any of my patients got better. If they did, I felt it was just luck.

This high failure rate was commonplace among the early practitioners, and it still is today among practitioners who have not evolved beyond that impaired system. Unfortunately, when myofunctional modality began to spread its wings, not much had changed, leading many practitioners and specialists to lose faith in it and unintentionally calumniate the science. It's no wonder myofunctional therapy often still gets a bad rap, especially from those who haven't taken the time to learn more about it.

Despite how narrow Ethan's jaws looked, his tongue could just fit up onto his palate, inside his upper teeth. I knew that it had the potential to exert expanding forces to widen the jaw. Hence, when he began wearing his mouthguard, I did not rush into constructing a removable jaw expander for him. The expander was in his original plan, but he was responding very well without it. Why would I make him wear a mechanical jaw expander when the myofunctional mouthguard was being effective? Trust the 'myo', as I would always say.

By the third month of wearing the mouthguard, the differences in Ethan's jaws, teeth, and bite were extraordinary. He still needed to practice a few exercises in between his monthly visits, but the mouthguard acted like his mouth's gym equipment. It was lifting his tongue up, pushing his cheeks away from the jaws, stretching his lips forward, and it was staying in every single night during sleep.

His swallowing had come a long way, with his tongue developing the ideal peristaltic wave motion. His cheeks and lips were not compensating for his tongue anymore. His lips remained closed in a relaxed manner at rest all the time. He was consistently breathing through his nose.

The domino effect carried through to his sleep. He had begun to sleep more deeply and for longer, waking up in the morning refreshed. His snoring had stopped, as his tongue would consistently be suctioning up against his palate, keeping his upper airway wide and patent. In other words, his body was receiving optimal balanced oxygenation, and his nervous system was regulated in parasympathetic. His sleep cycle had become optimized.

Ethan's progress with myofunctional therapy

Keep in mind that a myofunctional mouthguard is distinctly different from a mechanical jaw expander. The mouthguard works on the orofacial muscles, training them to posture and function better. When these muscles improve, they are the ones that place forces on the jaws and influence their growth and development. Then, when the jaws widen, the teeth have more room to position themselves into better alignment within the dental arches, positively affecting the bite.

In Ethan's case, he took full advantage of his mouthguard. His compliance was incredible. He did his exercises routinely, as instructed. I was ready to bet my house on it when I first evaluated him that he would need a mechanical jaw expander. I really did not see it coming, but everything about him was progressing beyond my expectations.

Do muscles always win?

CHAPTER 12 KEY FINDINGS

- A jaw expander can help when a child's growth needs an extra boost in a short time.
- The tongue is nature's own jaw expander – when it's strong and working well, it helps guide healthy growth naturally.
- It's not just about the tongue – the lips, cheeks, and other facial muscles all play a role, and they need to be supported together for the best results.

13

Cruising without turbulence

How the body and brain work together

It is not only about the muscles. Yes, they usually win against bones. What this means is that muscles exert forces on the bones and play a big role in shaping them. Nevertheless, the ways muscles function are controlled by how the nerves are firing and wiring.

Let's revisit the time when Ethan first came to see me. He was posturing his head and neck forward, likely having done so for many years. The dysfunctional breathing contributed to this poor posture. The tongue tie was also a causative factor not only for the posture but for the breathing itself.

As you have now discovered, the tongue tie is part of the fascia of the body, in particular the deep frontal line. This fascial line extends from the soles of the feet to the tongue, covering the diaphragm en route. The diaphragm is a breathing muscle. Its mobility can be affected if its fascia is restrictive, leading to dysfunctional breathing. If there is a tongue tie, there are likely other restrictive areas along this fascial line, including around the diaphragm.

The work that our team and Ethan's chiropractor did helped to loosen his fascial restrictions. Not only did his tongue improve, but so did his breathing and posture. All of this improved his functions, including the quality of his sleep. His diaphragm began to work during breathing, and he also began to improve his posture, especially of the head and neck.

Fascia tissues are also innervated by nerves. Poor postures and fascial restrictions can be related to the nerves not firing and wiring ideally. Take the vagus nerve, for instance. It is the longest cranial nerve that runs all the way down from the brain to our gut. It is a major part of the parasympathetic nervous system – your rest and digest.

There are two branches of the vagus that run along the sides of the neck. With forward head and neck posture, this nerve can often be irritated, as it gets bent or impinged due to the poor posture. Consequently, it may not fire and wire optimally; in other words, it may result in low tone. Having low vagal tone means the nerve's activity and responsiveness are reduced. When this is the case, it is difficult for the body to calm itself down from stress, which may lead to poor digestion, heart rate dysregulation, chronic inflammation, and emotional responses.

Have you ever come across a child throwing a temper tantrum in the middle of a supermarket aisle? In Australia, we refer to this as 'chucking a tantrum'. No matter how much the parent tries to reason with them, they just cannot stop. Sometimes they do it for so long that they cannot even remember why they're doing it in the first place. This child is in sympathetic overdrive, unable to get themselves out of the stressful situation. They are likely to have low vagal tone.

A few factors can cause low vagal tone – poor sleep, chronic stress, ongoing inflammation or illness, trauma, and even a sedentary lifestyle. The vagus nerve also plays a role in how we connect with others. It affects emotions, behavior, and physical health because our nervous system constantly shifts between calm and alert states, often without us realizing it. When stress becomes overwhelming, some people may shut down or withdraw. On the other hand, feeling connected to friends and loved ones can strengthen emotional resilience and help regulate the nervous system.

Yes, the vagus can be related to your social connections. My friend, Dr Genevieve Keating, a leading neurodevelopmental chiropractor from Melbourne, Australia, introduced me to the work of Dr Stephen Porges. He is an American psychologist and neuroscientist, who pioneered what is known as the polyvagal theory. He found that the vagus affects emotions, behavior and physical health, because our nervous system prioritizes survival by moving between the parasympathetic and sympathetic states, often unconsciously. People may shut down under extreme stress or trauma. Having friends and relationships may improve your emotional resilience, through connections and co-regulations. These are all associated with your nervous system.

Interconnected and not isolated

Interestingly, as you can see, I am back at how everything is interconnected. To me, it all feels like a destructive loop. But, does this mean we just need to intervene at the correct time and place to break the cycle? Well, it is not as easy as it sounds.

A lot of it comes down to whether you are able to find a practitioner who understands the interconnectedness. When you find one, that person will act like the director, pointing you down various paths, because they know they cannot work alone. And if you are the patient, you do need to be prepared to walk down these paths, particularly when you are determined to find the answers that you have been searching for for so long.

Sally was on such a journey. She knew that Ethan needed help, and needed it much earlier. Wherever she went, she found a roadblock. Nobody understood where to even begin. Not because they didn't want to, but because they didn't know. A serious problem facing healthcare in many parts of the globe.

When I went through dental school, we shared a few lectures with the medical students in our first year of the course. From the second year onward, we were separated. Our campuses were on opposite corners of a large intersection. The dental students were only taught about teeth and gums, basically. The only thing I knew solidly about the tongue was how to keep it out of the way so that I didn't nick it while doing a dental filling.

Functions were rarely discussed. No one mentioned how what we were doing in the mouth could affect other parts of the body. It felt like we were only working in such a special and isolated area, leaving us graduating oblivious about anything else. We came out of university as narrow-minded professionals with a fixed mindset, fearful of stepping outside our comfort zone.

Even within the dental school itself, the specialties interacted very little with one another. Almost everything was treated as an isolated issue. The education failed to train us to collaborate and integrate. Instead, it taught us only how to refer and let someone else deal with the problem. Yes, it's appropriate in some circumstances, but not in the majority.

The moment progress became visible

Five months into his treatment, Ethan would attend his visits with a smile on his face. He knew everyone in the clinic and greeted them all by name when he walked in. We gave him a bag at the start of his treatment to keep and carry his myofunctional tools and exercise instructions, and he would bring it with him every time.

His demeanor, stance, and gaze were all exuding confidence, calmness, and connection. I could actually have conversations with him, albeit briefly at any one time. From not being able to make eye contact to the person he was becoming – all he needed was to be given the keys. He opened the gate and took off.

Ethan's nervous system was regulating progressively. The tongue tie had gone. His fascia tissues were loosening and gliding over his muscles. These muscles were able to move like they had never moved before. His posture was more balanced, his breathing had calmed, and he was no longer snoring much during sleep. He was in cruise control.

Not only was Ethan now able to regulate beautifully between his sympathetic and parasympathetic states, but he was also socially connected. He felt like he belonged.

But because he kept thriving, the plan that I thought was strong and indestructible was actually being tested to its core. Strategizing my next move became a delicate balancing act between unpredictability and the unknown. I needed to take a step back and rethink my options. Everything seemed to be moving forward way too smoothly.

Was there something that I was still missing?

CHAPTER 13 KEY FINDINGS

- The nervous system has a powerful influence on how the whole body functions and responds.
- It can take time to find a practitioner who truly understands how everything in the body is connected – but it makes all the difference.
- When the right team works together to support your child's individual needs, their growth and progress can unfold more naturally and smoothly.

14

Breathing: the foundation of function

By the time Ethan had been wearing his mouthguard for three months, his jaws were widening, and his teeth were aligning well. He still had some degree of orofacial dysfunction, causing mild gaps between his upper and lower teeth when he bit them together, where his tongue would occasionally thrust.

I decided to move him to a second-stage mouthguard. It was firmer than the first one, keeping the cheeks and lips even further away from the jaws. He was to wear it for one to two hours every day while awake and every night to sleep. The orofacial myofunctional therapist prescribed him a couple of exercises for his mouth muscles to get used to the firmness of the device quickly.

The use of a removable jaw expander was still in the plan. I was not going to dismiss the possibility of using it yet. He kept proving me wrong, nevertheless. I was happy to be proven wrong on this occasion. His jaws continued to widen from his tongue optimally exerting forces onto his palate.

How muscles shape the face

As his upper jaw was developing, it was also freeing up the lower one. Gradually the lower jaw had more space to develop, widen, and translate forward. What was also helping this lower jaw to respond was that his tongue was functioning and posturing well. This meant that his lip, cheek, and chin muscles did not have to compensate for the tongue anymore.

Think about where the muscles of your face and mouth are located. First of all, the tongue is on the inside. It is attached to the lower jaw, but it needs to rest all the way up against the roof of the mouth. This elevated posture allows the tongue to exert forces on the upper jaw from the inside out. This supports ideal functions, such as breathing, swallowing, speaking, and so on.

The cheeks, lips, and chin are located outside the mouth, on your face. These muscles are resting against your jaws at all times. So, they do exert forces inward. However, if the tongue is not posturing and functioning well, the lips, cheeks, and chin need to work harder to help the tongue. When they work harder, they exert more force inward. For this reason, the jaws then receive heavier forces from the outside in than from the inside out.

Hence, when the lower lip and chin muscles are working harder, they contribute to holding the lower jaw back. An easy way to check this is by closing your mouth with your lips together and seeing if your chin is creasing, looking a little like a golf ball. If you can see the golf ball, it is likely that your chin muscle is under tension and unable to relax. This may be because it has been working harder than it is supposed to.

Add an open mouth posture into the mix. When the mouth is open, the cheeks are under tension, exerting more inward forces. The open mouth is usually associated with mouth breathing, in which the tongue has to sit low in the mouth. Yes, you got it! The jaws are unable to naturally widen because of this. Try it yourself. Open your mouth and feel the tension from your cheeks pushing inward.

Ethan had avoided needing a mechanical jaw expander or formal breathing retraining. His breathing was becoming calm and functional – through his nose, with his lips closed, and using his diaphragm instead of his chest. The simple breathing exercises prescribed by his therapist, together with fascial release and bodywork, made a remarkable difference. Not long ago, he had been a noisy mouth breather who couldn't keep his lips closed for more than a few seconds, constantly over-breathing and struggling to feel he was getting enough air.

Why good breathing technique is so important

The amount of air we breathe in and out is crucial for keeping the body's systems running smoothly. Oxygen is needed by every cell to produce energy, and without it, organs – especially the brain – can be permanently damaged within minutes.

Oxygen travels from the lungs through the bloodstream, carried by red blood cells containing haemoglobin. To reach the tissues, the oxygen must be released from the haemoglobin, and this depends not only on breathing itself but also on blood flow and how efficiently the oxygen is released.

A key player in this process is nitric oxide, a gas produced mainly in the nose and sinuses. It acts as a vasodilator, widening blood vessels to improve circulation and lower blood pressure. When we breathe through the nose, nitric oxide mixes with the air entering the lungs, enhancing oxygen absorption. Mouth breathing bypasses this step – meaning the body misses out on these benefits.

Carbon dioxide also has a vital role. It helps release oxygen from haemoglobin at the right time and place. The ideal level of carbon dioxide in the body is about 6.5%. If this balance shifts too high or too low, it affects blood acidity, which in turn impacts the brain and muscles.

My friend Dr Dan Hanson – a myofunctional dentist and Buteyko breathing practitioner – once explained this beautifully. Imagine a school bus taking students to school. The bus is haemoglobin, the students are oxygen, and the driver is carbon dioxide. Nitric oxide is the traffic controller, widening the roads to help the bus arrive on time. If you mouth breathe, you lose nitric oxide and exhale too much carbon dioxide. The bus keeps driving in circles, unable to stop and let the students out – so your tissues don't get the oxygen they need.

When this happens, the body becomes hypoxic – lacking oxygen. Fatigue, poor concentration, shortness of breath, and low coordination can follow.

Both gases do even more than this: nitric oxide supports immunity, brain signaling, and nutrient delivery, while carbon dioxide helps regulate blood pH, control breathing rate, and maintain healthy blood flow.

Breathe well, sleep well

Ethan had a tongue that could not rest or function up against his palate. It was tied down and sitting low in the mouth. When he slept, his tongue dropped back to narrow his airway. His mouth then needed to open as his body was not breathing sufficiently due to the tongue narrowing his upper airway. Fortunately for him, he did not have any other apparent obstructions in his upper airway, such as enlarged tonsils or adenoids. These would have made his breathing worse than it already was.

Even though he was mouth breathing during sleep, the upper airway was still narrowed by the collapsing tongue. So, he was snoring because the air going in and out had to pass through this narrowed tube, especially at the point where his tongue was obstructing. This led to his body 'waking up' multiple times in the middle of the night to regulate his breathing. Consequently, his sleep cycle was frequently disrupted, reducing his sleep quality and interrupting his body's repair and recovery phases.

The 'waking up' in the middle of the night did not mean he was fully awake and conscious. He could be moving around the bed constantly as his body needed to readjust and reinstate his breathing. The bed might end up messy in the morning as he would be restless all night long. In some circumstances, I have had patients experiencing night terrors that could be associated with having a breathing dysfunction.

People who mouth breathe tend to also have dry mouths, particularly upon waking up in the morning. This may result in a higher incidence of dental caries (tooth decay) and gum disease because of the lack of saliva cleansing and protecting the teeth and gums. The mouth becomes more acidic when it is dry, weakening the enamel of teeth and making them more susceptible to cavities.

Children who don't sleep well often wake up tired. You might notice dark circles or bags under their eyes – a sign that their blood circulation isn't working as well as it should. When a child is constantly overtired, their body and brain struggle to cope, which can show up in many ways, such as:

- becoming hyperactive or restless
- finding it hard to focus or pay attention
- showing sudden mood or behavior changes
- struggling to reason or think clearly
- shutting down quickly when they feel overwhelmed.

Think about how you feel after just one bad night's sleep – now imagine a child feeling that way every single day.

These are very similar symptoms to those of Attention Deficit Hyperactivity Disorder (ADHD). Up to half of children diagnosed with ADHD might actually have sleep-disordered breathing instead. This is alarming, in my opinion, because many patients diagnosed with ADHD have been prescribed medications that have possible long-term side effects. How many of them have actually been misdiagnosed when their issues were, in reality, their breathing health instead?

Breathing needs to be functional – that means closing your mouth, keeping your tongue up, using your diaphragm, and breathing through your nose. When your child practices this type of breathing, it can lead to:

- deeper, more restful sleep
- feeling refreshed and energized in the morning
- more stamina and focus during the day
- better stress control and emotional balance
- calmer behavior and improved concentration.

Ethan learned to do it – and your child can too.

CHAPTER 14 KEY FINDINGS

- It's not just about breathing through the mouth or the nose – what really matters is whether your child's breathing is functional or not.
- A healthy balance of oxygen, carbon dioxide, and nitric oxide helps the body and brain work at their best.
- The way your child breathes affects how well they sleep – and that sleep, in turn, shapes their growth, mood, focus, and behavior each day.

15

Are we there yet?

Looking before birth

Fascia. Nervous system. Breathing.

These are the three aspects of function that have so far been addressed for Ethan. These were his underlying issues, which led to him presenting initially with all the concerns he had. But what were the root causes? There were many possibilities, and it is difficult to pinpoint just one.

Ethan's older brother was also a patient of mine, as I mentioned at the beginning of this story. He did not have any of the concerns that Ethan had. He only needed simple orthodontic treatment to straighten his teeth and align his bite. His jaws were not narrowed. He did not have a tongue tie. He was breathing, chewing, swallowing, speaking, and sleeping well.

How, then, did two children from the same parents develop so differently?

I remember one particular occasion when a family came to see me for their oldest child. He presented with very similar concerns to those of Ethan. This boy was six years old. When he was born, his mouth was already open, with his breathing already noisy and effortful. His feeding was poor since birth. He had speech, eating, and sleeping issues. His parents could not work out what was happening, and they had been searching for answers.

What baffled them the most was that his younger sibling, who was born three years after him, did not have any of these problems. Feeding, eating, breathing, sleeping, and speaking were all fine. So, how could two children, born to the same parents, growing up in the same household, eating the same foods, and being raised in the same manner, have such contrasting functional development health conditions?

Our conversation during that first appointment felt like solving a mystery – one clue leading to another until the light bulb moment arrived. I asked the mother a simple question: 'Were there any differences between your two pregnancies?'

She paused, then shared that during her first trimester with her oldest child, her nephew had been gravely ill, and she had spent months supporting her sister through the ordeal. She was exhausted, fainted once, and often found herself mouth breathing and sleeping poorly. Her second pregnancy, by contrast, was calm and joyful. That realization brought the parents a moment of clarity – they could finally understand why their first child was struggling while their younger one was thriving.

The connection between pregnancy and childhood health

Nowadays, I tend to ask frequently about the health status of the parents when I see a pediatric patient. When a baby is growing inside the mother, all their systems are being shared. The mother is breathing, eating, sleeping, and exercising for two people. Hence, if the mother is hypoxic, the growing baby is likely to be in that state too.

Research has shown that poor childhood sleep is related to mothers who experienced less sleep duration during pregnancy. Mothers who had sleep-disordered breathing during pregnancy were associated with a higher risk of their offspring having congenital anomalies, especially affecting their musculoskeletal systems. Newborns of mothers who had obstructive sleep apnea were more likely to be admitted to the intensive care unit, requiring resuscitation and longer hospital stays. When the mother was highly stressed during pregnancy, the offspring were likely to have increased sleep problems in toddlerhood. Child sleep problems may have their origins in the fetal stage.

What kind of stresses might the mother experience during pregnancy? Psychological stresses, like the patient I saw above. Physiological stresses, like dysfunctional breathing and poor sleep. Environmental stresses, like being exposed to toxins and pollution. Lifestyle stresses, like working long hours and poor nutrition. Medical stresses, like chronic illness and substance abuse. There are many other stress factors that can impact the mother during pregnancy, which in turn affect the developing offspring in the womb.

From one generation to the next

Often these issues arise and get passed on to the next generations because of epigenetics. Epigenetics is the study of how behaviors, the environment, and external factors can cause changes in gene activity. The stresses mentioned above may alter the genes, which then affect the baby's genes, influencing possibly their future health and behaviors.

Epigenetics

It is clear that certain health factors can be inherited. I have even come across unexpected and prolonged post-release bleeding after a frenectomy, where the medical history of the patient appeared to be unremarkable. Further investigation revealed the patient was conceived with donor sperm. The biological father turned out to have haemophilia, a hereditary bleeding disorder, where the blood cannot clot properly due to a lack of certain clotting factors. From this incident, my team and I have added a question regarding how the baby was conceived to the new patient history form.

The difficulty arises when the medical histories of the biological parents are unknown. The practitioner and the parents may then get caught off guard when an unforeseen complication happens. In this kind of situation, it is favorable to remain calm and focused. Finding out the reason may take time, and a little bit of patience is much needed to resolve the issue.

As a parent myself, it is understandable to feel disappointed and even panicked in these circumstances. However, I do believe that all healthcare providers want the best possible outcomes for their patients. They are not out there to cause intentional harm, but complications do sometimes occur. Understanding the factors behind the events is key to rectifying the result.

Speaking of epigenetics, it is not impossible that the altered genes can be passed on over a number of generations. This is a concept known as transgenerational epigenetic inheritance.

In 1944 to 1945, a famine took place in the German-occupied Netherlands. The children of pregnant women exposed to the famine showed changes in the methylation of genes related to growth and metabolism. Some of these changes were also seen in their grandchildren.

Survivors of the Holocaust, or wars, had heightened stress responses, and their stress hormone regulation genes were altered. These genes were found in their children and grandchildren, likely due to inherited epigenetic changes.

Trauma can alter genes and then be inherited. Some of the offspring of those who survived the 9/11 attack were found to have similar reactions to loud airplane noises as their parents. These children were not yet conceived at the time of the attack.

It is mind-boggling to think that the root causes of many of our issues may have origins from generations before us. We are currently only scratching the surface of knowledge. There are plenty more layers of the onion to peel off. We are not there yet. We need to explore deeper and look closely into history. The puzzle is still missing several pieces, but when it takes shape further, maybe we can have a more solid direction on how to help our future generations.

CHAPTER 15 KEY FINDINGS

- Our genes can be influenced by our environment, lifestyle, and experiences – a process known as epigenetics.
- Changes in gene activity can sometimes be passed from parents to children and even grandchildren.
- Some health or developmental challenges in children may have roots that stretch back through previous generations.

16

Eat your veggies

The soft food problem

For muscles to build and bones to develop, exercising them is essential. Many children with narrow jaws lack the exercises needed to support the natural development of these structures. One effective and simple exercise is chewing.

We have discussed swallowing, but when we put food in the mouth, it needs to be chewed first before being swallowed. Chewing breaks down food for easier swallowing and absorption in the digestive system. In a sense, the mouth is our pre-digestive organ.

Ethan disliked certain food textures, mainly fruits and veggies. He was not chewing very much, as his preference was for softer types of food. A causative factor was that he found swallowing a struggle. The tongue tie had compromised his tongue mobility and swallowing. Hence, it was only natural for his body to choose softer foods, which he could swallow much more easily.

Unfortunately, soft processed foods have now been considered the norm in our modern society. Since the industrial revolution, especially, food has become more processed, manufactured in factories for effective distribution, convenience, and lower costs. Their nutrient content has decreased because they are made with artificial ingredients.

Have you ever had a crab stick before? Not exactly breaking news, but they are not made of crab meat. Instead, they are made of fish mixed with starch, artificial crab flavoring, sugar, salt, and coloring dyes to mimic the red of real crab meat. They are soft, requiring little chewing, making them easy to swallow. I see many children buying them at the fish and chip shops. Well, parents buying them for their children. Maybe it's time for us to stop and take a moment to think about what we are feeding our children.

Chewing builds strength

Chewing activates the muscles of mastication, which include the masseter, the temporalis, the medial pterygoid, and the lateral pterygoid. The forces of chewing are applied to the teeth and then to the jaw bones, developing these bones to withstand such forces, in turn.

Two of my friends, who strongly advocate globally the roles of chewing, are Dr Kevin Boyd, a pediatric dental specialist in Chicago, US, and Mrs Sharon Moore, an airway-focused speech pathologist in Canberra, Australia. Together, they have been spreading the message worldwide about the link between chewing and the growth of the jaws.

The side on which you regularly chew builds the bone thicker and wider. The bone on the side that you do not chew tends to grow longer and more vertical. Often, the way the teeth bite together can give us a clue as to which is the preferred chewing side of that person. When you look at the horizontal plane where the upper and lower teeth bite together from the front, it can be slanted when there is habitual one-sided chewing. The higher side of the slant is likely to be the preferred chewing side.

Another indication of one-sided chewing is when the palate is asymmetrical. The narrower half of the palate is usually the non-chewing side, as the jaw bone is not growing wider. This side also tends to have more crowding of the teeth, and the dental arch appears longer.

At the beginning of his intensive orofacial myofunctional therapy, the therapist gave Ethan a chewing silicone mouth tool. It fit inside his mouth like a mouthguard. His teeth sat in the channels of the device, where there were bristles that would stimulate the proprioceptive responses of his gums as he chewed.

'Ethan, I would like you to chew on this with your lips closed for 10 to 20 minutes a day,' the therapist taught him. 'You can break that up into maybe five minutes each session, as long as you reach the total daily chewing time.' He was not worried about it and inserted it as soon as he got hold of it.

When he first used it, we could all see how he visibly became calmer. It was as if he was able to regulate faster. What was occurring was that as he chewed, he produced more saliva in his mouth. He then needed to swallow more frequently. 'So whenever you need to swallow, Ethan, keep the mouthguard in your mouth and don't take it out to swallow,' the therapist educated him further.

With every swallow that Ethan did with the device in his mouth, sitting properly over his teeth, his tongue needed to push as high up as possible to perform the swallow. This would lead to the tongue pressing against the palate as much as possible, exerting forces to widen the jaw. If his cheeks, lips, and chin pushed in to compensate for the swallow, the mouthguard minimized the inward forces these muscles would exert on his jaws.

The exertion from the tongue would increase as Ethan continued to practice his exercises, and when his tongue tie was released.

What processed food has taken away

In the early 1930s, a Canadian dentist and researcher named Dr Weston Price traveled the world for about 10 years. He visited around a dozen traditional and isolated communities, including Swiss alpine villages, Gaelic communities in the Outer Hebrides, Native American tribes in North America, Inuit in Alaska, Polynesian islands, African tribal groups, Australian Aborigines, Maori in New Zealand, and South American indigenous groups.

His goal was to study the dental health, facial structure, and overall vitality of people eating traditional diets, especially compared to those who had adopted modern, processed foods. He found that people eating traditional, nutrient-dense diets had wide and strong jaws, straight teeth, virtually no tooth decay, and fewer degenerative diseases. In contrast, those consuming modern, industrialized foods (sugar, white flour, processed oils) showed dental crowding and decay, narrow facial structure, and increased disease and fatigue. He believed nutrition impacts not just the teeth but also mental health, immunity, reproduction, and bone structure.

The communities Dr Price visited were secluded from the modern world. They were hunters and gatherers, eating foods that required lots of chewing. They had their full sets of teeth with jaws wide enough to fit them all in without crowding. Their foods had not been tampered with chemicals and artificial substances, likely avoiding the risks of altering their functional wellbeing and genetic expressions.

Humans are naturally meant to have jaws wide enough to fit all their adult teeth. When the jaws grow properly, there's also enough space for the tongue to rest comfortably against the roof of the mouth, helping to keep the airway open. So, wide jaws aren't just about straight teeth - they're also key to healthy breathing and overall function.

Turning mealtimes into muscle training

Besides the chewing apparatus, we encouraged Ethan to eat more fibrous and crunchy foods. Using these foods to practice chewing can also be beneficial. 'How about having more raw carrot and celery sticks when you have lunch or dinner, Ethan?' I suggested to him. 'Just make sure that you chew using both sides of your mouth.' He was not really buying it initially, but Sally took on the idea and began including these in his meals.

Introducing solid foods to infants usually occurs at six months of age, when the first deciduous teeth erupt and the baby is developmentally ready. Baby-led weaning is one method that skips purées and spoon-feeding in favor of the baby feeding themselves. The baby is served real foods, which they can grasp, bite, and chew.

Not only does this approach promote their motor skill development, but it also encourages the baby to activate and use their chewing muscles effectively. Steamed carrots, broccoli florets, and whole lamb chops can be great options to feed them. Avoid processed foods and items that are small enough to become choking hazards.

Expect mealtimes to be messy, as they discover and build their interest in foods. Subsequently, they become more independent and confident with eating and eventually develop the skills to recognize hunger and fullness cues.

When food triggers inflammation

The kinds of foods we eat can also make a difference. There are three main food groups known to be more inflammatory to humans: refined sugars, pasteurized dairy, and gluten. I have seen many patients who are sensitive or intolerant to these foods, with the most common symptom among them being congestion, affecting airway health and breathing functions. Sometimes the tonsils and adenoids become enlarged.

Sometimes parents choose to try an elimination diet to see whether certain foods are affecting their child's health. This means removing the suspected food for about four weeks and making sure it isn't accidentally eaten during that time. If the food really is a trigger, parents often notice that congestion eases or even clears up completely, helping their child breathe and sleep more easily.

Of course, not everyone is sensitive or intolerant to the food groups mentioned above. An assessment by a nutritionist, a naturopath, or an integrative medical doctor can be useful in evaluating individual reactions to foods. These professionals can also assist in formulating meal plans that suit the needs of each person. Seeing an allergist might be needed if an allergy is suspected. Allergy testing can clarify uncertainties and help in determining what to avoid.

The ancestral diet

My preference is to follow the ancestral diet. It refers to the way humans ate before the rise of industrialized, processed foods.

Fundamentally, it encompasses what our ancestors consumed for thousands of years across various cultures and environments. It's not actually one specific diet, but rather a set of principles based on traditional, whole-food eating patterns that support long-term health, fertility, and resilience.

The core principles of the ancestral diet are:

- **Whole, unprocessed foods** – no refined sugars, flours, seed oils, or synthetic additives. Foods are eaten as close to their natural state as possible
- **Animal-based nutrition** – organic meats, fatty cuts, bone broth, raw dairy, pastured eggs, seafood, and animal fats like tallow, lard, and butter
- **Nutrient density** – focusing on foods rich in fat-soluble vitamins (A, D, K2), minerals, and essential fatty acids
- **Fermented and cultured foods** – sauerkraut, kefir, yogurt, fermented fish, and miso for gut health
- **Preparation techniques** – soaking, sprouting, fermenting, and slow-cooking to enhance nutrient availability and reduce anti-nutrients
- **Seasonal and locally sourced** – eat what's available locally and seasonally, not what is available all year round
- **Avoid industrial seed oils** – no canola, soybean, sunflower, or corn oil. Replace them with traditional fats like butter, ghee, coconut oil, and olive oil.

At the end of the day, you are what you eat. Every bite is a choice to heal or harm yourself. Food is one of the most powerful medicines you can take. Having real foods will give your body fuel to achieve real results.

CHAPTER 16 KEY FINDINGS

- Chewing is nature's way of strengthening your child's jaw, face, and airway – it's just as important as exercise for the rest of the body.
- Many modern foods are too soft, which means kids aren't using their chewing muscles enough to grow strong, healthy mouths.
- Focus on real, whole foods that your family enjoys – the closer to nature, the better for long-term health and development.

17

From the top down

'I look like I've had braces already.'

Ethan took to the second stage mouthguard like a champion. He wore it for at least one hour daily while he was awake. It stayed in all night, every night, while he was asleep. He practiced his exercises twice every day.

His jaws were widening and growing forward as his orofacial muscles progressively improved. Because the jaws were developing favorably, his teeth were all moving into place accordingly. As it happened, his teeth were aligning into a Class I dental occlusion, meaning that the upper and lower teeth are biting in an ideal relationship. This Class I dental occlusion is what orthodontists aim for when treating patients with dental crowding.

Ten months after commencing his treatment, his orofacial functions and postures were as optimal as he could get them. As you can see from the progress photos, his jaws and teeth improved significantly. He did not need mechanical jaw expansion devices. He did not have any extractions of adult teeth. He did not have orthodontic braces or clear aligners.

At that 10-month visit, I asked Ethan what he thought about his teeth. I pointed out that some of his side teeth were not exactly locking into his bite yet. These might continue to improve, or he could have braces or clear aligners to fine-tune their positions. He said to me, 'I look like I've had braces already.' Well, he was not wrong.

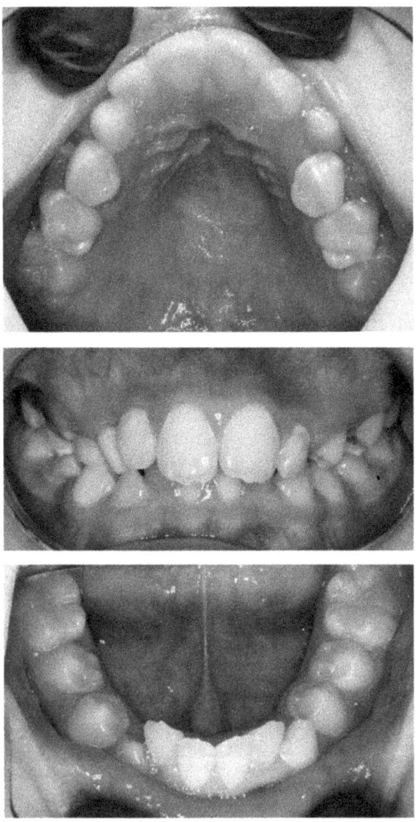

Before treatment.

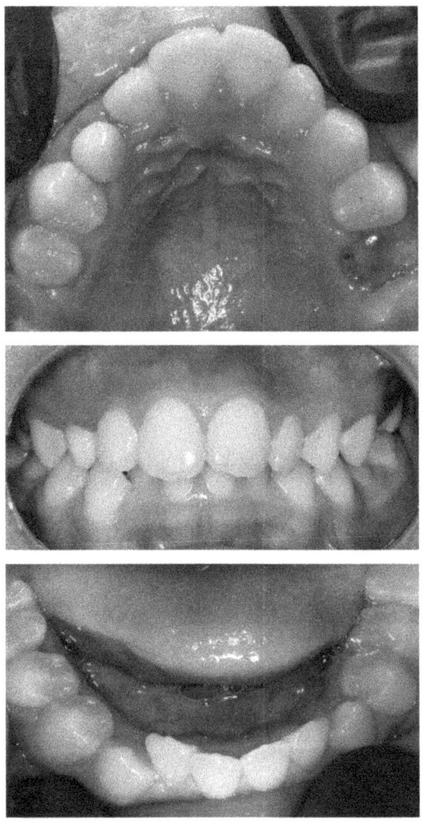

Two months into treatment.

Collaboration and shared learning

Vital to Ethan's successful outcome was the collaborative approach. I did not look after him alone. The orofacial myofunctional therapist was heavily involved. His mother was an integral part of the team, especially for his compliance. And one consequential member of his team was the neurodevelopmental pediatric chiropractor.

The mouth is part of the face. The face is part of the head. The head sits on top of the neck, which connects all the way down the body, through the shoulders, hips, knees, and to the feet.

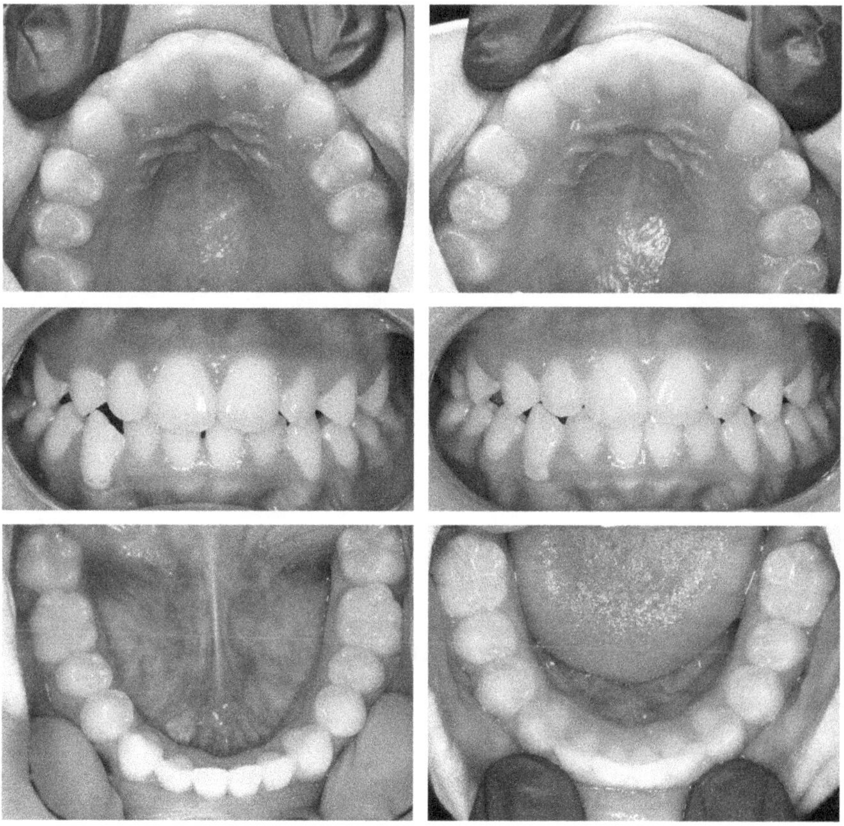

Five months into treatment. *Ten months into treatment.*

Chiropractors and osteopaths play essential roles in assessing and managing the patient's postural, fascial, nervous, and cranial systems. As a dental practitioner, my scope is to remain within the boundaries of the head and neck, with a focus on the mouth.

I do feel it is important for me to understand how the entire body works with all its interconnected systems. For this reason, I have gone out of my way to study further from clinicians outside my field. I have so far learnt from chiropractors, speech pathologists, lactation consultants, ENT (ear, nose, and throat) specialists, nutritionists, kinesiologists, physiotherapists, and osteopaths.

In mid-2025, I attended a comprehensive cranial osteopathy course and workshop in New York. Out of the 52 students, only five were dental practitioners. The rest were osteopaths. I found this very interesting, because I thought all osteopaths would work the same way. No, as it turned out. Many osteopaths have not been taught about cranial osteopathy in their university degree and need to seek further education for it after they have graduated.

Chiropractors are in a comparable situation. Some of them pursue specialized training in Sacro-Occipital Technique (SOT), which is somewhat similar to cranial osteopathy. And some pursue further learning in neurodevelopment, focusing on the development of the brain and the nervous system of children, from newborns onward.

Come to think of it, we, dentists, are actually in the same boat. I have not found a dental school, in Australia at least, that teaches about orofacial myofunctional science. Only a few of us understand how the functions of the muscles of the mouth and face are related to how these structures are going to form. Quite astonishing, considering this science has been around for more than 100 years.

The head-body connection

The cranium is the skull. It is made up of eight bones. The jaws are part of the facial skeleton, which attaches to the cranium. Therefore, evaluating and managing the cranium are crucial when the jaws are being treated, because they are linked to one another.

Cranial bones enclose and protect the brain. Inside this cranial cavity, there are also meninges (protective membranes), the cerebrospinal fluid, blood vessels, and the cranial nerves, besides the brain itself. They all need to work together for healthy development of the brain. By age six years, the brain has reached approximately 90% to 95% of its adult size, signifying the importance of supporting its growth as early as possible.

From the cranium and down through the entire body, there is a subtle rhythmic motion that is independent from breathing. This concept is known as the primary respiratory mechanism (PRM), which is central to osteopathic cranial philosophy. It is believed to play a defining role in overall health and functions.

The main components of the primary respiratory mechanism (PRM) are:

- inherent motility of the brain and spinal cord – the brain and spinal cord have a natural, rhythmic expansion and contraction
- fluctuation of the cerebrospinal fluid (CSF) – this fluid circulates rhythmically, contributing to the movement of the cranial bones and the dural membranes
- mobility of the intracranial and intraspinal membranes – the dural membranes (protective layers that protect the brain and the spinal cord) move in rhythm with the PRM, helping to transmit motion throughout the central nervous system

- articular mobility of the cranial bones – the cranial bones are not completely fused and can undergo subtle rhythmic motion at the sutures (joints)
- involuntary mobility of the sacrum between the iliac bones – the sacrum (base of the spine) moves in coordination with cranial motion via the dural tube connecting the skull and sacrum.

Imbalances or restrictions in the PRM can contribute to headaches, jaw joint disorders, stress, tension, sleep disorders, postural imbalances, and even infant feeding or developmental issues. PRM imbalances are believed to result from mechanical, postural, muscular, or developmental factors that affect the cranial bone mobility, dural membrane tension, cerebrospinal fluid fluctuation and sacral alignment.

If we break down these causative factors, they can be grouped as follows.

1. Cranial trauma or head injuries

These can affect the mobility of cranial bones, sutures, or tension in the dura mater. For example:

- birth trauma (forceps delivery, vacuum extraction, C-section)
- falls or blows to the head
- concussions or whiplash injuries
- dental trauma or orthodontic invasive interventions.

2. Spinal or sacral dysfunction

These can impact the reciprocal tension membrane system via the dural tube. For example:

- misalignments in the sacrum (for example, sacroiliac joint restriction)

- spinal injuries or poor posture
- falls on the tailbone.

3. Abnormal breathing patterns or airway restrictions –

These conditions may alter cranial base motion or pressure dynamics affecting PRM. For example:

- chronic mouth breathing
- obstructive sleep apnoea
- deviated nasal septum or enlarged adenoids and tonsils
- the tongue collapsing back to narrow the pharyngeal airway.

4. Muscle tension or fascial restrictions

These can influence the mobility of cranial bones or the sacrum through connective tissue continuity. For example:

- tension in the jaw (temporomandibular joint (TMJ) dysfunction)
- tension of the neck or facial muscles
- myofascial restrictions in the head (tongue tie, lip ties, cheek ties), neck, or pelvis.

5. Developmental or birth factors

These can affect early cranial bone movement and dural membrane tension. For example:

- positioning of the baby in the womb (for example, breech)
- long or traumatic labour
- premature birth.

6. Emotional or psychological stress

Chronic stress may lead to increased muscle tensions, especially in the neck, jaw, and diaphragm, which may restrict craniosacral rhythm and dural flexibility.

7. Dental or orthodontic work

Braces can impact the motion of the upper jaw and associated cranial bones. Tooth extraction or jaw joint misalignment can affect bite, muscle tension, and cranial base balance.

8. Infection or inflammation

Meningitis, encephalitis, or chronic sinus infections can disrupt the cerebrospinal fluid flow or cranial bone mobility.

Untangling cranial strains

The positions and relationships of Ethan's jaws when he first presented were likely to also be associated with his cranial health, to some degree. The base of the cranium is the floor of the cranial cavity. This base can become distorted or strained, especially due to trauma, such as birth trauma, or developmental reasons, such as the positioning of the baby in the womb.

Strains of the cranial base influence the positions and relationships of the cranial bones and can be associated with cranial asymmetry and facial asymmetry in all axes. Consequently, because the facial bones are closely related to the cranial bones, the positions and relationships of the upper and lower jaws are affected by these cranial strains.

With Ethan, his lower jaw was retruded, meaning that it was trapped and positioned too far back. It was locked in this position partly due to one of his cranial strains. This presentation is common in people with a hyperflexion strain of the cranial base. In hyperflexion, the lower jaw, which is related to the cranium through the jaw joints sitting against the temporal bones, is 'pulled' back due to these temporal bones being rotated outward.

I believe that everyone has some degree of cranial strains. Having multiple strains is expected. Besides influencing the jaws, these strains can also affect the activities of the cranial nerves, muscle functions, and posture.

In my opinion, I doubt that cranial strains can be permanently fixed, especially in individuals with no growth potential. They can be improved and stabilized, and the patient requires regular maintenance from a qualified cranial bodyworker. Nevertheless, with improvements and stabilization alone, I can see that the growing patients are reaping functional benefits from these.

Why jaw work starts at the head

I have had patients needing mechanical jaw expansion devices who required routine cranial bodywork. These appliances work directly on the upper jaw, commonly aimed at widening and growing the jaw sideways and forward. Because the upper jaw is directly related to the cranial bones, I have had patients with cranial locking (reduced, or even no cranial mobility) who did not respond well to the expansion therapy. If the cranial bones are locked, it is more difficult for the upper jaw to move. These patients may experience headaches or sometimes feel generally unwell if their jaws are repeatedly mechanically expanded. Basically, the upper jaw is being pushed against the skull, which cannot move.

The tongue is nature's best jaw expander. When it presses up against the palate, it helps guide the jaws to grow wide and balanced. But if the cranial bones are tight or restricted, the jaws can't always respond properly to the tongue's efforts.

For this reason, simply widening the jaws mechanically isn't always the answer – especially for adults. It's important to first understand why the jaws are narrow and make sure the body is ready before starting treatment. If the underlying issues aren't addressed, the body may stay stuck in its old compensation patterns.

Cranial therapy can help by gently improving movement through the skull and fascia. These practitioners support the nervous system, release tight tissues, and help the body work as one connected system. In my view, they're an essential part of any team that's supporting healthy growth and development.

CHAPTER 17 KEY FINDINGS

- The jaws and the skull grow and move together – what happens in one can influence the other.
- When the jaw or head is out of balance, it can affect posture, breathing, and overall development.
- Working with a skilled cranial bodyworker helps support healthy growth by gently aligning the head, jaw, and body as one connected system.

18

Integrating reflexes

Have you ever come across a child who cannot pay attention and stay focused? A child who is clumsy, bad at reading and writing, and has poor posture? A child who is bedwetting beyond the typical age? A child with delayed milestones, like crawling and walking? This child may have retained primitive reflexes.

I have come across many of them in the clinic and even outside of my practice. A knowledgeable and skillful bodyworker can often help them to integrate these reflexes.

Primitive reflexes

Primitive reflexes are automatic movements that babies are born with – built-in survival mechanisms that develop even before birth. They help newborns feed, move, and adapt to life outside the womb. Doctors can observe these reflexes during pregnancy and after birth as signs of healthy brain and nervous system development.

As a baby's brain matures, these reflexes should naturally fade – usually within the first year. When they don't, it may indicate delayed or atypical neurological development. Retained reflexes can interfere with movement, posture, balance, attention, learning, and behavior. They can also contribute to issues such as clumsiness, poor coordination, or even bedwetting (often linked to the spinal galant reflex).

Children with ADHD, autism spectrum disorder, sensory processing disorder, dyslexia, dyspraxia, or developmental delays commonly show signs of retained primitive reflexes.

Failing to integrate

Why do primitive reflexes sometimes fail to integrate? The reasons may be biological, environmental, or neurological. Birth trauma or difficult labor may be causative, as they can affect the infant's nervous system and disrupt natural movement patterns essential for reflex integration. Premature birth may lead to incomplete activation and integration of in-utero developmental milestones.

Lack of movement may limit necessary sensorimotor experiences. Babies need specific movements, like rolling, crawling, creeping, and tummy time, to develop their motor pathways and integrate these reflexes. Spending too much time in car seats, baby swings, walkers, or bouncers prevents them from experiencing natural movements.

Prenatal exposure to stress may also result in failure to integrate as it interrupts brain development. These stresses can include the mother getting infections, illnesses, or emotional strains. Drugs, alcohol, and environmental toxins are also antagonists. Underlying genetic disorders or brain abnormalities can also affect the integration process.

Why integrate?

Many of the new patients presenting at my clinics would arrive bouncing off the walls. They looked like they had just had a big sugar hit. Some had, but some had not. Others arrived looking lethargic, with bags under their eyes, pale skin, and shoulders slumped down and forward. No matter how they presented, they had usually never been assessed or managed by an appropriate bodyworker. Their nervous systems would be highly dysregulated, leaving them in a state of sympathetic overdrive, or they had been sleeping so poorly that they were exhausted. For these patients, listening and following instructions would be almost impossible.

There were occasions where I would recommend that parents not proceed any further at that point in time, because their children were simply not ready. The last thing I would want is for parents to waste their effort, energy, time, and money.

Most of the treatment that my team and I implement requires compliance, with some ability for the patient to listen and follow instructions. Yes, the treatment itself can help improve these abilities. However, if their body does not allow them to do so in the first place - because they have a dysregulated nervous system or retained primitive reflexes - then these issues need to be addressed before anything else.

Although outside my scope, I do have the skills to observe possible retained primitive reflexes when I see them. I do not usually diagnose them, because I am not qualified to do so. This is where the appropriate bodyworker comes in.

Integrating these reflexes involves specific physical exercises that support brain development. Repetition is key. The movements are designed to mimic early developmental patterns, helping the brain and nervous system complete their developmental processes. It is about taking the brain back to infancy and retraining it to inhibit reflexes that should no longer be active.

Integration sessions need to be short and regular – around 10 to 20 minutes each. They should begin at the neurological and physical levels of the patient, whether a child or an adult. Starting slowly is usually best. Integration is a neurological process, and patience is necessary. These sessions need to be guided and managed by qualified professionals such as a neurodevelopmental chiropractor, cranial osteopath, or occupational therapist.

Come to think of it, integrating primitive reflexes sounds very similar to orofacial myofunctional therapy: begin with simple exercises, do not overload the patient, repeat and repeat, be consistent, then progress gradually when the patient is ready.

Ethan had poor posture when I first met him. He still needed to wear night nappies, or diapers, until he was about nine years of age. He had many contributing factors to these issues, as we have discussed so far. Another likely factor was that his primitive reflexes were not yet integrated.

Thank goodness he went to see the neurodevelopmental chiropractor. Over time, these reflexes began to integrate as he continued his treatment with us. I could not help thinking that his demeanor, mannerisms, and behavior all changed partly because of this.

CHAPTER 18 KEY FINDINGS

- Babies are born with natural reflexes that help them during birth and support their growth in the first year of life.
- If these reflexes don't integrate when they should, they can affect how a child moves, learns, functions, and behaves as they grow.
- Working with a skilled bodyworker can help gently retrain the brain and body so these reflexes integrate properly.

19

Ah-choo

The case of the unexpected sniffles

I once had a patient who completed his treatment with my team and me when he was eight years old. He was initially a mouth breather, causing his jaws to narrow due to the lack of palatal forces from his tongue. Through orofacial myofunctional therapy and preorthodontics, he got better. His habitual mouth breathing progressively turned into functional nasal breathing. His sleep quality improved, and he began to wake up feeling refreshed regularly. He used to need at least a couple of dental fillings every six months, but that changed too.

After he completed his active treatment, he would return every six months for me to monitor his natural jaw growth. He would wear his myofunctional mouthguard every night to sleep to maintain his orofacial postures, which supported his jaw development. He had photos taken at every visit so that we could analyze the changes.

He returned every six months for a couple of years. Because he was stable and his growth was heading in the correct direction, his maintenance visits were then extended to once a year. His mouth-guard actually needed to move up in size, as his jaws widened steadily.

When he was 14 years old, he presented for his annual maintenance visit. I was shocked. He had dark circles under his eyes. His breathing was noisy, with his mouth open. He was congested, sounded nasal, and had a runny nose.

'What happened?' I blurted.

His mother was heartbroken. She seemed lost. 'It all started three months ago,' she answered. They went to the doctor and were told that he was just sick. But he never got better. His sleep was worsening again; he began to snore and also grind his teeth. The nights would now be restless, and he would wake up as if he hadn't even slept all night.

I could easily see that his tongue was sitting down low again in his mouth. His gums were red, looking dry from the mouth being open most of the time. The myofunctional device was not staying in at night anymore. 'It's quite funny,' he said. 'I woke up one day a couple of days ago, and our puppy got hold of it. It must have fallen off the bed. I think he thought it was a toy!'

A puppy? It suddenly occurred to me that this could be the reason. As it turned out, they welcomed a puppy into their family ... you guessed it ... three months ago! I knew I was onto something here. But my head was spinning at the same time. How was I supposed to break the news that he could be allergic to the dog?

Would I suggest getting rid of the puppy? Of course not!

When breathing feels hard

One of the most common concerns I hear from patients is feeling like their nose is always blocked. When this happens often, it usually points to a chronic issue - most commonly allergies or exposure to environmental irritants - leading to ongoing inflammation. While inflammation is part of the body's healing process, if the cause isn't addressed, it can linger and overload the immune system, affecting both breathing and overall function.

Inside the nose are nasal turbinates, which filter, warm, and humidify the air we breathe. These can become enlarged from allergies or infections, making the nose feel constantly congested. The nasal septum - the wall dividing the two sides of the nose - can also bend if space inside the nasal cavity is limited. Because the floor of the nose is the same bone as the roof of the mouth, a high palate or narrow upper jaw can reduce nasal space, contributing to congestion and restricted airflow.

Ultimately, the nose and mouth form one functional unit. When the upper jaw doesn't grow wide or forward enough, it not only limits space for the tongue but also narrows the airway. My friend Dr Jeevanan Jahendran, an internationally renowned ENT specialist from Kuala Lumpur, Malaysia, always asks, 'Is the elephant too big for the room, or is the room too small for the elephant?' In most cases, it's not that the tongue is too big - it's that the room it lives in is too small.

When an ear, nose, and throat specialist is needed

Ear, nose, and throat (ENT) specialists are experts in evaluating and managing the upper airway. They understand the associations between upper airway volume, breathing functions, sleep quality, and craniofacial development. Many of them collaborate with dentists because of this.

A knowledgeable ENT specialist attempts to find the root cause of upper airway issues. The tonsils, adenoids, and nasal turbinates become enlarged for a reason. Removing these inflamed structures may provide immediate short-term relief for breathing and sleeping, but without identifying the causes of their enlargement, removing them may not be effective in the long term.

Nevertheless, ENT specialists can assist in improving upper airway volume by reducing obstructive inflamed structures, commonly through the use of nasal hygiene protocols, anti-inflammatories, or surgical intervention. Those who have a deeper understanding of the interconnectedness may collaborate with nutritionists or naturopaths to address possible dietary causes of the inflammation, bodyworkers to address the nervous, fascia, and lymphatic systems, breathing educators to address breathing, orofacial myofunctional therapists to address myofunctional issues, sleep physicians to address sleep quality, and even allergists to address possible allergies, and dentists/orthodontists to address jaw development.

If the patient has suspected allergies, a referral to see an allergist may be required. The patient may not be aware of having allergies. These allergens can be dust mites, pollen, grass, foods, medications, insect stings, mold, or even pet dander (just like with my patient).

I remember another patient of mine whose parents witnessed him having sleep apnea episodes during sleep, where he was holding his breath and gasping for air regularly. He was severely congested constantly, and they could not find the reason. Until one day, they sought the services of a building biologist, who found a hidden mold infestation under the floor of his bedroom. They renovated and cleaned it all out, and his sleep improved almost immediately.

Allergies, sensitivities, and intolerances can impact functional health unknowingly. The affected patient can worsen without realizing what is actually happening to them.

Ethan, fortunately, did not suffer from allergies. His tonsils and adenoids were not obstructive. He did not frequently become congested. I did not feel he needed to have an assessment with an ENT specialist. His upper airway was compromised, nevertheless, because of his tongue collapsing back into it and his craniofacial complex development being inadequate.

It was a different story with my other patient, who was allergic to dogs. He went to have tests done by the allergist, and the results confirmed my suspicion. Because giving up the dog was not an option, he underwent immunotherapy, which gradually trained his body to tolerate the allergen. Over time, this would reduce or eliminate the allergic reactions. It took him quite a few months to eventually be able to play with his dog. He was thankful that he got to keep ... Sniffle.

CHAPTER 19 KEY FINDINGS

- Allergies are a common reason children struggle to breathe well – and they can be tricky to identify and manage.
- Keeping the nose and airway open and clear is essential for healthy, functional breathing.
- Enlarged tonsils, adenoids, or swollen nasal tissues are often a reaction to something else – not the root cause of the problem.

20

It ain't over till it's over

Genetic potential: unlocked

In ten months, Ethan was able to achieve positive changes that I never thought would be possible. His age, underlying medical conditions, and social challenges were all working against him. Everyone he saw declined to give him a chance until his mother brought him to see me.

There was something in him that bestowed a glimmer of hope. He was seeking hands that would help and guide him, without even understanding what he was really looking for. Deep down inside, he was a fighter, refusing to give up. It was not easy for him to recognize the emotions he kept hidden inside for so long.

Sally, though, kept an open mind. She was determined to search for and find the oasis that she always knew existed. Every time I saw her, I could feel how proud she was of Ethan. Her eyes would light up and her smile would broaden whenever he achieved a goal. He achieved many goals in that short amount of time.

It was all about unlocking his own unique genetic potential. One that had been suppressed all his life, eager to be set free. Only the right timing, the right place, and the right team could turn the key and unlock the gate. Once it had been opened, he did not turn back. Ethan took it and ran.

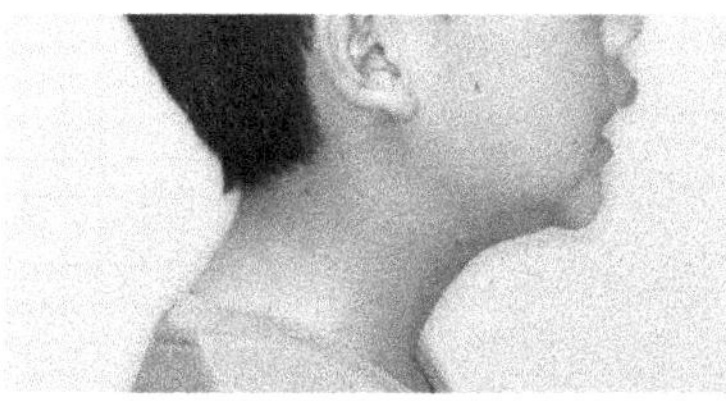

Before treatment.

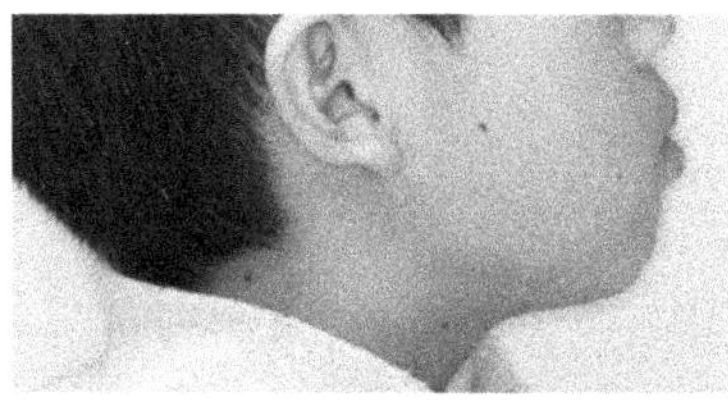

Two months into treatment.

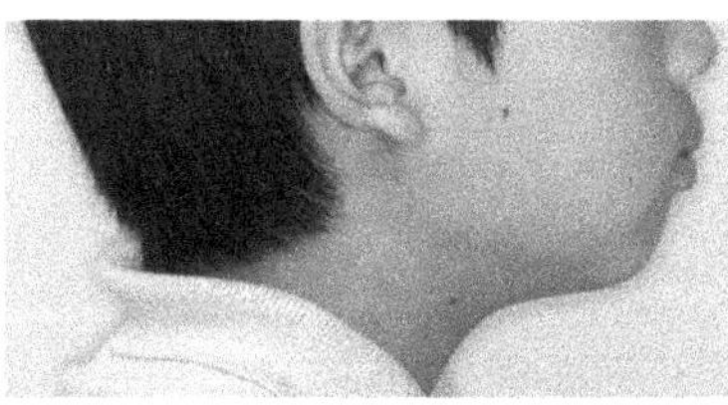

Five months into treatment.

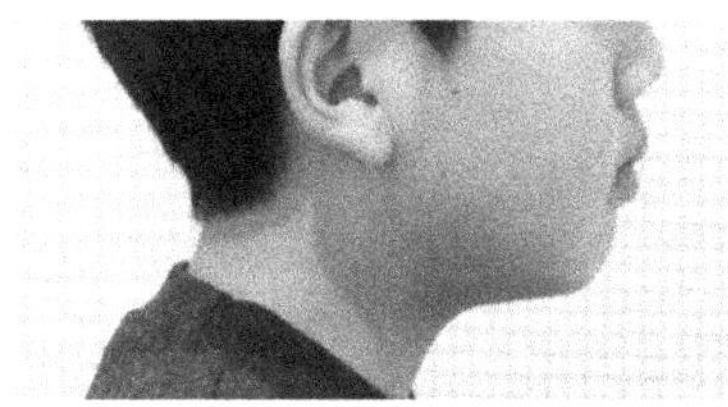

Ten months into treatment.

At his last active treatment appointment, I prescribed him the third-stage mouthguard. It was the firmest of them all. Designed to provide retention and maintenance, it was to be worn every night until his natural growth and development had completed, at 18 years old at the very least.

His mouth and face muscles were functioning as well as they could. He had established an elevated tongue posture, with the entire top surface of his tongue resting against the palate. His lips were closed at rest, without strain from other facial muscles trying to keep them together.

When Ethan was breathing, he was quiet. He was not using his chest to breathe anymore. The amount of air going in and out through his nose was controlled and balanced. He did not need to posture his head and neck forward to keep his upper airway patent. His diaphragm was free to fulfill its role in functional breathing.

To ensure his orofacial functions and postures remained stable and supportive of his craniofacial growth, the therapist reminded him to be mindful of his tongue, lips, and breathing at all times. By this stage, these postures and functions should already be habitual and automated neurologically. But it's still better to be safe than sorry.

Do not lose it

There were three things he needed to practice whenever he felt like his mouth and face muscles were regressing.

The first was suctioning and holding his tongue all the way up against the roof of his mouth. 'Now Ethan, it is not just the tongue tip, but the entire top surface of the tongue. Like super-gluing the entire tongue to your palate. Then, stretch it by slowly opening your mouth as wide as you can without dropping the tongue down,' the therapist reminded him. When he looked in the mirror, he could see two caves under his tongue, left and right, with his tongue attachment separating them down the middle.

This tongue suction hold and stretch exercise would retrain Ethan's entire tongue to elevate all the way up. It would increase the tone of his tongue muscles and strengthen them to remain in the elevated position. Consequently, he would not be able to breathe through his mouth when his tongue remained glued to his palate, as it would be sealing the oral cavity from air being able to enter and exit.

When your child's tongue rests up against the roof of the mouth, it helps calm and regulate their body by stimulating the vagus nerve. This supports healthy hormone balance, better recovery from stress, and steady growth. The gentle pressure of the tongue on the palate also helps the upper jaw widen naturally, giving space for the lower jaw and teeth to align into a stable, healthy bite.

The second was swallowing properly, where the tongue would do all the work, with no compensations from other muscles of the mouth and face. With this mature swallow exercise, there should not be movements from the cheeks, chin, head, and even the eyes while performing the swallow. 'Remember to do this in front of a mirror, Ethan,' the therapist suggested, 'so you can see if any part of your face is moving or not. Try to make sure nothing is moving except for your tongue.'

When food or liquid sits on the tongue, the lips should be closed to form a seal. The tongue tip then pushes up against the roof of the mouth, moving the bolus backward. This creates a wave-like motion as the tongue continues to propel the bolus toward the throat. As the swallow is about to occur, the teeth clench for a second or two, and the epiglottis (the valve in the throat) closes over the trachea (windpipe), preventing the bolus from entering the respiratory tract. The digestive tract then continues the wave motion that began with the tongue, carrying the bolus downward.

During swallowing, the tongue alone should exert upward forces against the palate. Other muscles around the face and head should remain relaxed. If the cheeks, lips, or chin need to compensate for a dysfunctional tongue, these muscles will pull inward, restricting the natural growth of the jaws beneath them.

The third exercise Ethan needed to remind himself of was silent belly breathing. This meant having his lips closed together at all times while inhaling and exhaling through his nose. His breaths needed to be slow, small, and shallow, as his diaphragm would be pumping the air in and out of the lungs, not his chest doing the work.

This would be useful whenever he found himself opening his mouth to breathe, which would indicate that he was over-breathing. By that stage, he was fully aware that oxygenation of his organs needed to be optimal, and over-breathing would be detrimental to this process due to the excessive loss of carbon dioxide from his system.

Through nasal breathing, not only would the air get filtered and humidified, but he would also carry nitric oxide into his circulatory system. The benefits of this particular gas would then be fully utilized and realized. All three gases involved in breathing would then find their ideal balance to serve their purposes.

Ethan nodded to accept the challenge. He knew the game plan had changed. It was not about playing catch-up anymore, but about keeping it all at the rate and direction that they were supposed to continue along. He seemed relieved that the hardest part was behind him. What he achieved was truly remarkable, and even Sally was amazed at how far he'd come.

But this was not the end – he continued to baffle us.

CHAPTER 20 KEY FINDINGS

- When your child's natural potential is unlocked, their body begins to grow and develop the way it was always meant to.
- Once orofacial postures and functions have been optimized, they need to be maintained so that they become automated and habituated for that person.
- The key goals to support healthy growth are simple: tongue up, lips closed, functional breathing, and a mature, natural swallow.

21
The endless puzzle of parenthood and health

Have you ever tried to solve a jigsaw puzzle that felt like it was never going to end? It said 1,000 pieces on the outside of the box, but when spread on the table, there seemed to be a million.

Finding a piece that fit with another was an achievement. After every one, you would run around the table for a victory lap. Then back to the struggle and frustrations. Slogging it out bit by bit while doubting if this was all worth the effort.

And when the big picture started to take form, slowly and surely, everything began to make sense. The pieces had always been there all along, staring right back at you. Even the box gave it away. Yes, the picture had been on the box all this time. All you had to do was reproduce it by connecting the parts correctly. Sounded way too simple, but not quite so in action.

Yet, during the tussle, there would be times when you would lose faith. Giving up would cross your mind a few times. Should you fall into this temptation? It would probably be much easier if you had not started it in the first place. Not knowing would be the uncomplicated option.

Seeing the whole picture

Through many years of learning, studying, and treating, I believe the more I know, the more I realize how much I don't know. This jigsaw puzzle of functional health seems like it will never be solved. There are more and more pieces coming up to the surface, which provide reasons but instill further complexity. The human body is one intricate unit that can easily break down with one wrong move. But its determination and will to survive often mask the cracks.

Interconnections are everywhere. There is an abundant amount of information out there, being released at record speed. Health providers are sharing what they know from every corner of the globe. Often, things can become quite overwhelming. How many practitioners do I need to take my child to see to get them to thrive?

As a parent, I see the other side of this dilemma. There is very little time each day to fit everything in. And yet, we still, of course, strive to do our best for our children.

The way modern societies have been evolving and are heading toward is concerning for everyone. It is all about convenience. How quickly can we get things done? Ready-made meals. Online shopping. Delivery to your door. Streaming services. Social media. Let's just stay home, binge on shows, and not move. I am not surprised that functional issues, behavioral disorders, and chronic diseases are prevalent.

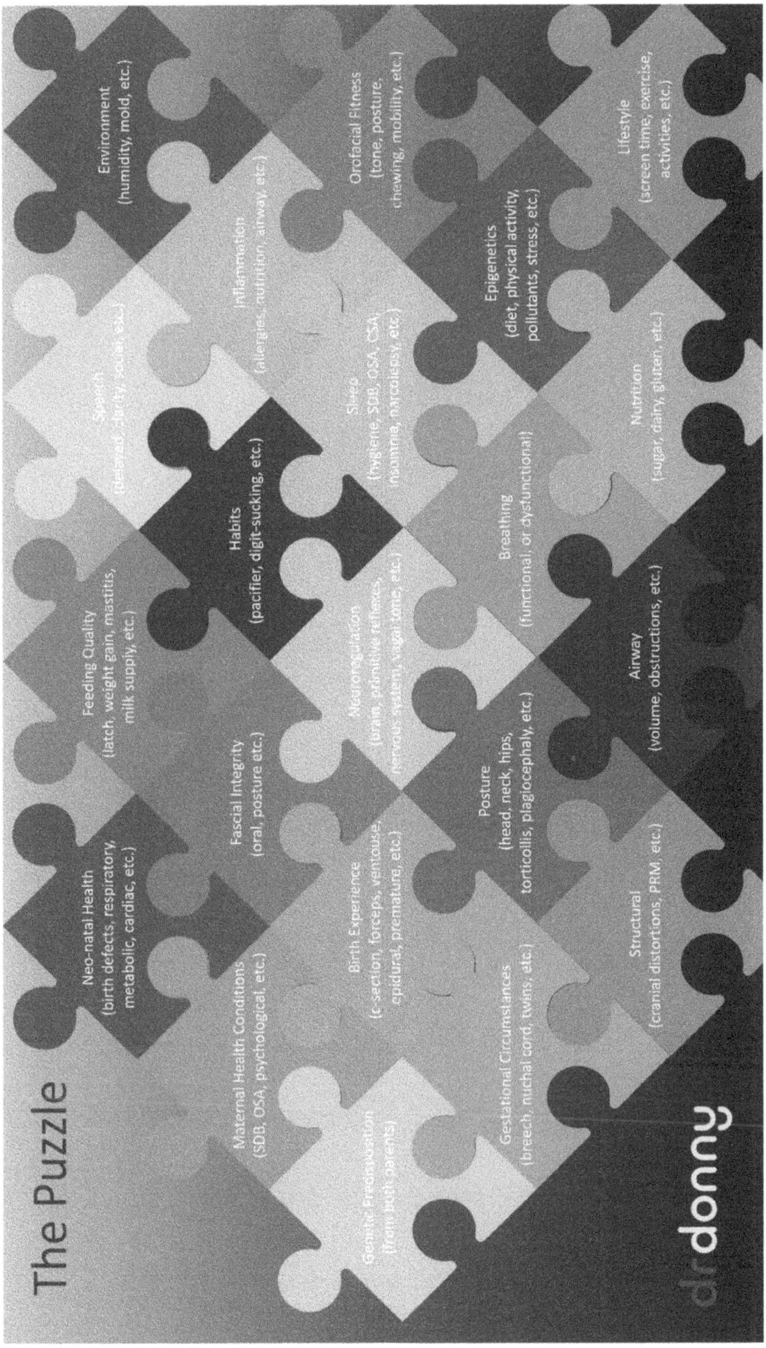
The Puzzle
Neo-natal Health (birth defects, respiratory, metabolic, cardiac, etc.)
Feeding Quality (latch, weight gain, mastitis, milk supply, etc.)
Speech (delayed, clarity, social, etc.)
Environment (humidity, mold, etc.)
Maternal Health Conditions (SDB, OSA, psychological, etc.)
Fascial Integrity (oral, posture etc.)
Habits (pacifier, digit-sucking, etc.)
Inflammation (allergies, nutrition, airway, etc.)
Genetic Predisposition (from both parents)
Birth Experience (c-section, forceps, ventouse, epidural, premature, etc.)
Neuroregulation (brain, primitive reflexes, nervous system, vagal tone, etc.)
Sleep (hygiene, SDB, OSA, CSA, insomnia, narcolepsy, etc.)
Orofacial Fitness (tone, posture, chewing, mobility, etc.)
Gestational Circumstances (breech, nuchal cord, twins, etc.)
Posture (head, neck, hips, torticollis, plagiocephaly, etc.)
Breathing (functional or dysfunctional)
Epigenetics (diet, physical activity, pollutants, stress, etc.)
Structural (cranial distortions, PRM, etc.)
Airway (volume, obstructions, etc.)
Nutrition (sugar, dairy, gluten, etc.)
Lifestyle (screen time, exercise, activities, etc.)
drdonny

The jigsaw puzzle of functional health.

It is very common to see children at restaurants, on screens the entire time, while their parents are actually having conversations. I even see younger couples on dates where they are both fixed on their phones. On that note, I used to need to work hard to ask someone to go on a date. Nowadays, you just swipe left or right, and you don't even need to engage in real conversations anymore.

What is this world turning into?

Be the free thinker

The puzzle of functional health keeps growing, with countless factors shaping each person's story. The root cause of an issue can start even before conception – and continue to build through pregnancy, birth, and childhood development. Every child is unique – even siblings raised in the same home can have entirely different outcomes, just like Ethan and his brother.

The key is to keep learning and stay open-minded. Step beyond your comfort zone, question assumptions, and learn from every experience – especially from your children. They often teach us more than any textbook ever could.

Be the free thinker that I have been advocating for.

Gathering the right team

Finding the right open-minded person to help you is another challenge. Not all health practitioners can think outside the box. I do find that word of mouth is the best avenue to find that person. Don't be afraid to share your story with your friends and family. They may be able to direct you down the road you have been searching for.

Then, when you are on that road, the person you first feel connected to can be the one you appoint as the director. The one who can guide you and build the team you need around you. This director can be the myofunctional dentist, the cranial pediatric osteopath, the neurodevelopmental chiropractor, the speech pathologist, or even the ENT specialist.

Once you have a team you are comfortable with, make sure that each team member is communicating with the others. The team designs, plans, and executes the entire program. They all need to have the same goals in mind and remain on the same page at all times. There is no point in going in circles and getting lost, as this creates confusion, which limits the achievable outcome to a lower level.

Trust and believe in the process. Yes, there will be many appointments to make and fulfill, but with progress, things do get easier. With growth, everything takes time. There is no such thing as a quick fix. The initial steps need the most attention while working to get the patient as close to the law of nature as possible. After that has been accomplished, it is all about nurturing what nature intends to do.

Strong foundations

When you open that can of worms, one thing after another keeps revealing itself, taking you deeper and deeper. However, never forget your intentions. These are the foundations of why you are in this rabbit hole in the first place. The foundations give you the base and strength to build upon so that the finished building does not easily sway or crumble away.

In Kyoto, Japan, there is a temple that was built in the year 778. It is a massive edifice sitting on top of a timber cross-sectional substructure, where not a single nail was used. Not a single nail. Yet, it has stood the test of time.

Humans are built in a similar way. In every aspect of our lives and bodies, we need a strong foundation to begin with. By having such, any problems that we encounter along the way will become more straightforward to deal with. We all face problems as we live, and how good we are at facing them depends on how stable and strong we are deep inside.

But as I have mentioned a few times throughout this book, we are all individuals, and none of us are exactly the same. Hence, there is no recipe book that we can go by. There is no one-size-fits-all type of prescription that can cure everything. As a matter of fact, this substantiates the significance of having that sturdy framework to begin with.

Stepping beyond the comfort zone

Despite how far we have come in learning about whole-body functions, the majority of health practitioners still hold traditional beliefs and values. They only know about structures, and most of them do not actually want to know anything else. The excuse is usually that they are waiting on the research. Well, there is plenty of evidence available. If you are not aware of it, that does not mean it does not exist.

I used to fall into that category. Tertiary-level education taught us to stick to the recipes, as they have been proven to work. Treating a patient according to a step-by-step instruction manual is not about healing – it is more about putting a band-aid on.

When I graduated from dental school, I wanted to be a prosthodontist – a specialist in prosthetic dentistry, such as dental crowns, bridges, and implants. I even went on to obtain my fellowship in implantology. As I treated more and more patients, I continued to question why and how they ended up in this state. What journeys had they been on that led them to develop dental cavities, break teeth, and sometimes lose teeth altogether? Placing prosthetic dental materials was not treating the root cause. I was only fixing and restoring them.

Then a few of the dental implants I placed would sometimes fail. They would not integrate, or fuse to the jawbones. Back then, it was only reasonable for me to think that my surgical technique needed to improve. I kept blaming what I thought were my own poor technical skills. I was supposed to solve the problem for my patients right there and then – that was the expectation of a dentist every single time. If you could not solve the problem, then you were not a good enough dentist.

Looking back at those patients whose dental implants failed, I began to see a pattern. They all had dysfunctional breathing. Their mouths were always open. Their jaws were narrow. Their faces were long. They were always tired and would complain about how stressful their lives were. I never asked them about their breathing, their sleep, or their functional histories back then. I was oblivious to all of that. Now I have realised that they were chronically inflamed and neurologically dysregulated. Their bodies were under constant stress, contributing heavily to the failures of the treatment I performed.

Of course, I cannot rule out the possibility that my technical skills were suboptimal – it is definitely a feasible reason. But I could not have been that bad, as many other patients I treated did not experience such failures.

There is nothing wrong with staying inside the box. Ethan and Sally met a few of those practitioners before they came to see me. Some of them are actually among the very best at what they do – and we need them. If I, for instance, had an accidental knock and broke a tooth, I would definitely need to see a typical general dentist who could fix it for me.

They remain in that box because that is where they feel comfortable. There is no need to rock the boat or venture into the unknown. They know what they know. They do not know what they do not know.

As for me, I want to know more. The frightening bit, though, is that as I learn more, I feel like I know less. It is like a puzzle that does not want to be solved. Pieces keep appearing, and the search has no end in sight. The world of functional healthcare has only scratched the surface. In a few years' time, my puzzle will truly be made up of a million pieces.

CHAPTER 21 KEY FINDINGS

- Every challenge your child faces usually has more than one cause – it's rarely just one simple thing.
- Helping your child reach their full potential starts with building strong, healthy foundations.
- Working with a practitioner who looks at the whole picture – and understands how everything in the body connects – can make all the difference.

22

What waits beyond

Never stop learning

I am still hungry for more. There are no boundaries to how much you can learn, as long as you have the desire to keep doing so. It is the only way, I believe, that I can continue to serve my patients.

Through the years, my treatment protocols have evolved on a number of occasions. After all, change is the only thing constant in this world. Thus, I strongly believe that no one needs to be afraid of change.

Sometimes a course of treatment needs to change because of unforeseen circumstances. Or, maybe, because something new has come to light and will be more effective in helping the patient out. Evolving as you continue to serve is surprisingly doing yourself and the patient a favor.

With progress, what I am now capable of is on an entirely different level to what I was like when I first became a dentist. This translates to better care for my patients. Healthcare that is more comprehensive, holistic, and integrative.

And so, would I have managed Ethan differently if I met him today? Maybe, or maybe not. It's difficult to say, as my team and I looked after him in the best possible way we could, based on the knowledge and skills we had then.

Photobiomodulation

Nowadays, I am releasing fewer tongue ties. Not everyone needs to go through the experience of having a tongue tie release procedure, if they don't absolutely have to. There are some tongue ties that do not need to be physically released. They may only need fascial adjustments and exercises from the orofacial myofunctional therapist and the bodyworker. And if the tongue attachment feels tight, but there is no functional impact whatsoever, do we still need to surgically release it?

A technological advancement that I have been studying is the implementation of photobiomodulation therapy, specifically using low-level laser machines. This therapy can help in reducing inflammation, stimulate healing, and relieve pain in tissues. It is called low-level laser because it can penetrate through skin and the deeper layers without actually 'cutting' them. The technology has been around for quite a while, and you may have come across it for various applications, like muscle recovery, hair growth, and skin rejuvenation.

The kind of low-level laser that I am referring to, however, is not the one commonly used. It is more penetrative, to target the fascia, loosening tightness around the neck, face, and inside the mouth. Therefore, if the tongue tie is located more toward the base of the tongue, this therapy alone may be sufficient to decrease the restriction, without the need for a surgical release procedure. It does not replace the retraining exercises, though, as these are still necessary to improve the organ's strength and tone. In other words, the non-invasive low-level laser helps the patient to be able to retrain the orofacial muscles more easily.

This is something that can be beneficial for patients of any age group, when there are fascial restrictions present. With infants, for example, sometimes when they are struggling to breastfeed, it does not always mean there are ties inside the mouth that need to be surgically removed. They may have restrictions that can be loosened using this technology instead.

On that note, from what I have seen, having bodywork on infants from a pediatric cranial osteopath or a neurodevelopmental chiropractor may already be enough to improve the breastfeeding experience. In a way, low-level laser therapy complements the treatments from bodyworkers.

Craniodentology

Speaking of bodyworkers, my understanding of the cranial system has also expanded. I, or anyone, cannot deny that the jaws are connected to the cranium. Hence, when I am treating the jaws for them to grow and expand, I need to take into account what the cranial bones are doing. If there is locking of the cranial system, it is unlikely that the bones are going to respond due to the lack of mobility.

Having the knowledge of how the cranial system works can also help me in determining if the cause of the problem is located somewhere else in the body. The head and the tailbone (sacrum) are connected anatomically and functionally by a core link. This is made of dural membranes that cover the brain and the spinal cord, which extends all the way down to the sacrum, transmitting motion between the two areas. For this reason, if the sacrum is locked, there is a likelihood that the cranial locking originates from way down the line.

Another facet where an association is likely to exist is to the eyes. The trigeminal nerve is the largest of the cranial nerves. This cranial nerve V has branches to the upper and lower jaws, and also to the eyes. Dysfunctions of the jaws may irritate this nerve, causing potential eye and vision issues. On top of that, muscle tightness, or fascial restrictions, can also contribute to symptoms around the orbits, such as pulling sensations around the eye, tired eye feeling, and pain when moving the eye, despite the eye itself being healthy. Collaborating with behavioral optometrists is already taking place.

To look after my patients holistically, I need to recognize all possibilities. This does not mean that I am qualified to treat the issue directly, especially when it originates from outside my areas of scope. Nonetheless, if I can at least make the observations, I am able to fulfil my role as the team director more effectively. Consequently, the patient will be the one reaping all the benefits, as doors are being opened for them to get closer to their ultimate destination, by being managed by practitioners that they actually need.

Three dimensions

As the knowledge and the treatment options are widening, the tools of evaluation need to be able to move along with them. Although my clinics are well equipped with all the latest in technology, the hurdle of being able to maximally utilise them is often due to bureaucratic reasons.

Three-dimensional computed tomography cone beam (CBCT) machines are a supreme tool in producing X-ray images of the patient's craniofacial structures. From the scans, measurements can be generated for the jaw sizes and positions, the upper airway volume, the symmetry of the bones and jaw joints, and so on.

Because of the pediatric nature of my practices, the brand and model of the CBCT machines that I installed were chosen with the utmost considerations. These particular machines are designed to minimize the radiation exposure as much as possible, while still producing the optimal image quality.

According to the manufacturer, the reduction of radiation is up to 52.6%, compared to conventional CT machines. They also only take 2.9 seconds to capture the images, instead of 24 seconds with the conventional machines.

This low-dose technology, which is safer for patients, has been available for a while. Yet, there are people in positions of authority who have been preventing my team from taking advantage of them to their maximum potential. These are ones who do not understand fully that we do prioritize the safety of our patients, while remaining comprehensive in our care.

Professional respects

Yes, I am frustrated, and I apologize for venting. My point of bringing this up is to demonstrate that being progressive and a few steps ahead can end up in a position of scrutiny. I do feel like I have a target on my back.

The example above is about a machine. However, there are professionals out there who are going out of their way to intentionally halt progress by being vocal about concepts and philosophies that they do not actually comprehend. It is unfortunate when these things are being said, coming from a point of bias.

My patients all need to see their general dentists for their oral health. I don't know many of these dentists and have never heard of even their names before. They have never met me, nor listened to any of my presentations. Surprisingly, some of them have told some of our mutual patients that what I do is a sham. They are happy to claim that there is no science behind it, without even taking the time to read and learn about it. I find these situations to be very sad.

Is it just ego, or are they afraid of losing their market share? Just to be clear, myofunctional dentistry is not about avoiding braces or clear aligners. These are treatments that may still be needed to align and straighten the adult teeth. The purpose of intervening early is to take advantage of the natural growth potential while it is still high. If you can recall back to chapter 1, the face has completed 80% of its natural growth by the age of six. So, does it make sense to wait?

What I would like my patients to avoid is having jaws that are narrow. The narrow jaws result in insufficient room for the tongue and reduced volume of the upper airway, including the nasal passages. If the adult teeth are crowded because the jaws are narrow, extractions of some of these teeth may be required, especially if the treating practitioner is only concerned about how straight the teeth look, without considering the functional health of the patient. The fewer teeth present in the mouth, the smaller the jaws become.

This is not about trying to compete with other dentists and orthodontists for profits. In fact, working together with orthodontists is the preferred situation. We focus on the orofacial muscles and fascia, while they focus on the teeth. The harder part of the entire treatment paradigm is actually the functional therapy. Moving and aligning teeth are much simpler to perform when you do not need to 'fight' against dysfunctions.

When we graduated from dental school, we all had to take an oath, which framed our ethics as we went out to practice. The main intention was to make sure that we do no harm. That's no harm to patients and to our colleagues. Our pledge was to remain safe, moral, and to carefully consider all aspects of what we do for the sake of the communities that we're involved in.

As a matter of respect, I believe in learning both sides of the story, before even sharing my own personal opinion. There is no advantage in giving my two cents' worth, or even worse, to disparage someone or something, with no solid basis underpinning my action. We need to embrace progress. Stalling it will only handicap humanity.

Somehow, hearing about the negativity tends to be the one leaving a more lasting effect in the mind. Thankfully, the majority of my colleagues do hold similar beliefs as me. It is a rarity, to be honest with you, to come across ones that do not.

I am grateful that my patients are seeing the results with their own eyes. They are my advocates, who have experienced the benefits of early intervention myofunctional dentistry themselves. I witness the lives of their children, themselves, and their families being continuously transformed, on a daily basis. This brings me the sense of accomplishment and joy, as it validates the importance of the work we do as a team.

Subsequently, my patients are my driving force to keep moving forward. The more people we can help, the greater the chance we have for the future generations to achieve optimal functional health. Because of them, continuing to evolve and advance is a necessity. They are the ones telling the story, which hopefully will carry on to amaze all of us.

CHAPTER 22 KEY FINDINGS

- Not every tongue tie needs to be released.
- New technologies and research are continuing to emerge, providing more non-invasive healthcare options.
- Progress is often limited when practitioners are unwilling to look beyond a narrow perspective.

23

The end of the beginning

As Ethan was walking out from the practice, at his last active treatment visit, the cold winter clouds cleared to reveal the bright blue sky. The wind was still chilly, but the warm rays of the sun gave us the sense of comfort and relief. He walked upright with his chest forward, oozing a whole lot of confidence that he did not have almost one year prior. He smiled and thanked all of us. We could all see how proud he was of what he had accomplished.

Sally was equally cheerful. She was immensely appreciative of the teamwork that we managed to form around her son. The result was beyond her expectations, as she was led to believe by those they saw before me that it was going to be impossible. The possibilities turned out to be endless for Ethan.

I was in awe myself. The trust that I had in nature was already strong. Yet it surprised me once again. Compared to the initial plan I formulated for Ethan, there were a number of steps that he successfully avoided. He did not need dedicated breathing retraining therapy, nor the mechanical jaw expansion appliance, nor the fixed braces, the clear aligners, and the jaw surgery.

When his post-treatment X-ray was compared to the one he had before he commenced treatment, it was evident that both his upper and lower jaws had grown forward. This translated to not only more space for his tongue to posture and function optimally inside his mouth, and his teeth having enough room to align, but also for his upper airway to remain wide.

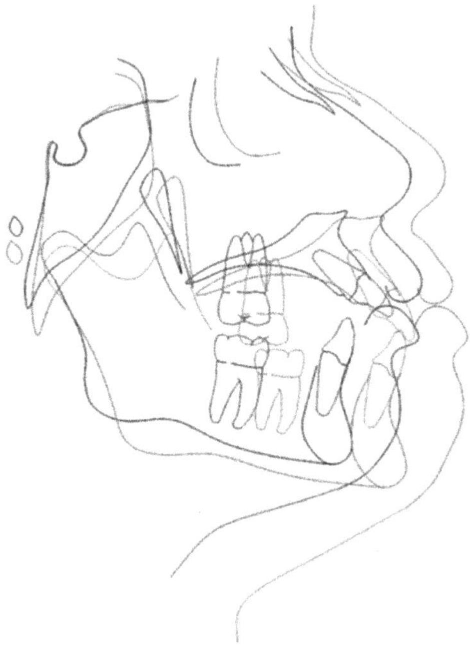

Superimposed tracings of Ethan's X-rays. Black lines are before treatment and grey lines are after treatment.

It was not goodbye, however, because Ethan would still need to return once to twice a year, to have his natural jaw development monitored. Until he's at least 18 years old, he would need to wear his myofunctional mouthguard to sleep every night, to continue to maintain his orofacial postures as these muscles would support and encourage his jaws to grow in a favorable direction. The mouthguard would need to be changed once in a while, because of wear and tear, and also size increases due to his continuous jaw growth until maturity.

A journey together

You have by now been on a journey alongside me and the team that Ethan had. Together, we have discovered the roles that genetics, epigenetics, the nervous system, the cranial system, the fascia, the muscles, nutrition, the environment, movement, breathing, and sleep play on functional health.

When all of these need to be taken into consideration, it does sound and feel overwhelming. Remember though, that this does not mean every factor calls for a dedicated practitioner for the patient to see. Your days do not have to be constantly filled with appointments.

A myofunctional dental practitioner can look after the orofacial functions and jaw development. A cranial osteopath, or a neuro-developmental chiropractor, can look after the nervous system, the cranial system, the fascia, and the posture. An ENT specialist can look after the airway and sleep. These are only examples of a few providers, to illustrate the multi expertise of each profession. There are many more that may need to join the team, such as speech pathologists, lactation consultants, nutritionists, pediatricians, orthodontists, physiotherapists, integrative medical doctors, and others.

Between each profession there are overlaps in what we can do. The director of the team is the best person to suggest which specialties are essential to join the team. This does not also mean that the team has to remain the same throughout. The team needs to be dynamic, prepared to keep up with the changes that the patient makes as they progress with the treatment. Each member of the team needs to understand that new team members may be added and existing ones may be excused accordingly. Even the director needs to keep an open mind about this.

It is wonderful to see progress during treatment. A congruent team expects this from their patient. Progress translates to improvements, where the patient is becoming healthier, as their unique genetic blueprint gets unlocked. And if because of the progress a provider's job is done, it is a successful outcome.

Personally, I would like to let my patients go knowing that they are going to continue to flourish without needing me much anymore. Their goals are met and their enhanced functions become automated and habituated as part of their normal. When their normal is their optimal, then you can safely say that they have reached their maximum potential.

Maintaining nature

Six months after his final active treatment visit, Sally brought Ethan back to have his first review appointment. Up until then, he continued to wear his myofunctional mouthguard every night to sleep, with it staying in all night until the morning when he would wake up. He was seeing the neurodevelopmental chiropractor still, regularly every few months, for similar maintenance purposes.

Ethan was a lot more engaging by that stage. He remained very familiar with the clinic, and remembered where everything was supposed to go. He could hold conversations with a lot less effort.

There was no more avoiding eye contact. Sally did not have to speak on his behalf.

His jaws continued to develop in the right direction, because his orofacial functions were stable in their optimal conditions. He was breathing soundly, sleeping well, and eating better than he had ever done before. His adult teeth had all erupted into their ideal positions, creating a bite that was functional and healthy.

It was very obvious to see that Ethan was flourishing.

At his second maintenance visit, where half a year had passed since his last, he began to really come out from his shell. He was close to becoming a typical teenager. I noticed that even his fashion sense was changing.

He told me that he loved wearing his mouthguard every night. He felt lost without it. Unsurprisingly, he continued to maintain his normal at his optimal level. And so, his lips were always closed together at rest. There were no apparent compensations to his functions. His nervous system was firing and wiring with ideal connectivity.

I prescribed him a new mouthguard, because of wear and tear with his existing one. He was excited. He could not stop admiring how shiny it was in the emerald green color it came as. It was like getting the latest version of his favorite toy. There was no difference to his old one, except that it was in pristine condition.

The next visit for him was then scheduled for 12 months later.

These maintenance visits become further apart when the patient stays compliant and on course. The automation and habituation of the functions are established when there are no signs of regression. Be mindful of external forces that may alter the direction of growth. Recall the boy who was allergic to his dog.

Not only while growing, but even when we are not, having regular maintenance is never a bad idea. We use our bodies 24 hours a day. The systems are always going through the cycles of working and recovering.

How long do we drive our cars each day? Definitely not for the entire day. Yet, they need servicing every 6 to 12 months, because some parts may need to be repaired or even changed, usually from wear and tear.

Our bodies need servicing too. We cannot live without them. If they break down then we are in trouble, and likely to become incapacitated. I, myself, have periodic adjustments from my chiropractor, and also my osteopath. Fine tuning and recalibrating the parts provide better longevity. We put our bodies through a lot on a daily basis.

One year quickly passed by. It felt like I only saw Ethan last week, when he returned for his next maintenance visit. The appointment was in the middle of the pandemic that the world was navigating through at that time. He was not affected though. He went on with his routine and kept his functional health intact.

The myofunctional mouthguard was in excellent condition. It would sit in his mouth passively, where his orofacial muscles would posture and work around it. These muscles were so accustomed to the device. They were happy and content.

Ethan's jaws and teeth continued to improve. They were solidifying their placements and relationships. His wisdom teeth were the only ones unerupted by this stage. They were not going to erupt until between 18 and 24 years of age. The size of his jaws indicated that he was in a really good position as he was approaching the final phase of his natural growth.

The punchline

For some reason, three years went by before Sally brought Ethan back. Life got in the way. Not difficult for this to happen. When they returned, I had relocated my clinic to a new location. Bigger and better, I would like to believe.

As soon as they arrived, Ethan could not contain his excitement. He greeted everyone at the front desk. He asked for my retired receptionist by name, and was sad to hear that she was no longer working there. He was ecstatic to see my other receptionist and assistants again, nevertheless. He remembered everyone's name.

The energy in the place lifted. There was this young man, smiling broadly, saying hello to every person he met. Other patients could not help but notice him, and were instantly cheered up by his vibrancy.

He saved his greatest joy for my therapist and me. He could not wait to show off his teeth and jaws to us. He enthusiastically reported that he was wearing his mouthguard every single night. He knew that he had done well, and he was not afraid to show how proud he was of himself.

We updated his photos and compared the incredible changes to what he was like before treatment. Sally could not wipe the smile off her face. She repeatedly thanked us, but we extended our appreciation to her and Ethan. They were the ones who did all the work. Every member of his team was present to merely guide them and empower them with the tools he needed. Without Ethan and Sally, there would be no team.

Ethan was thriving without limits. Yes, he was still on the spectrum. However, he had blossomed into a person full of life. He defied the odds and left the non-believers to fend for themselves. His onion had been completely peeled off. The core had been uncovered from under the many layers that were keeping it hidden.

All he needed was to be given the chance and not be turned away. He grabbed the opportunity and never looked back. His puzzle was the closest to completion that it had ever been. Every piece found its match, and the picture was taking shape as he marched on.

I gave him a hug as he was about to leave. Sally then turned around and stopped him from walking away. 'Wasn't there something you wanted to tell Dr Donny before we go?' she prompted him. Ethan paused and thought for a quick second. 'That's right! I almost forgot,' he proclaimed. Then he whispered to me his news. My jaw dropped open, my eyes welled up, and my heart was filled with pride.

Ethan got his driver's licence!

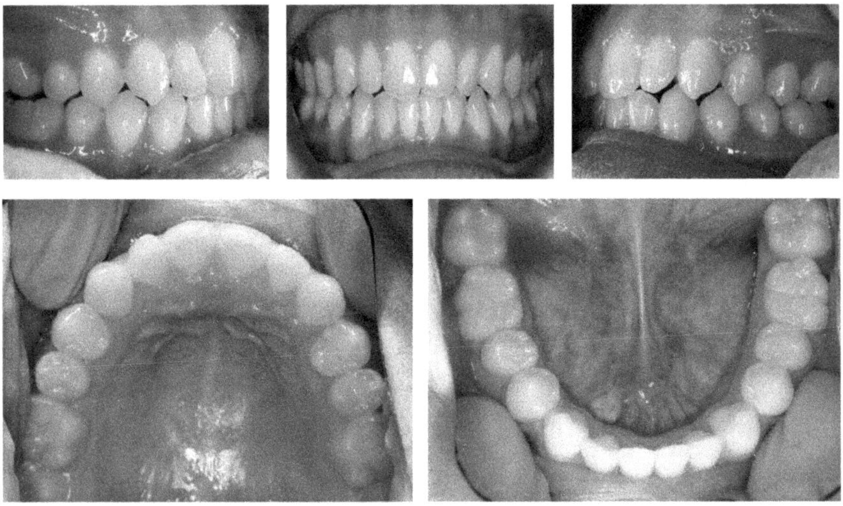

Ethan's jaws, teeth and bite, five years after completing his active treatment.

Growth never stops

Growth never stops. The more I learn, the better I serve my patients. My treatment protocols have evolved constantly over the years, shaped by new knowledge and changing circumstances. Each shift – whether prompted by necessity or discovery – expands my ability to deliver more comprehensive, holistic care. Looking back, I know my team and I have always done our best with the tools and understanding we had at the time.

Today, my approach is gentler and more precise. I perform far fewer tongue tie releases, recognizing that not every restriction needs to be cut. When function isn't truly impaired, therapy and muscle retraining can often achieve the same result. One of the most exciting advances is photobiomodulation, or low-level laser therapy. This light-based treatment reduces inflammation and pain while stimulating healing, helping loosen tight fascia and supporting other bodywork techniques – often sparing infants and children from unnecessary surgery.

My work now embraces the whole cranial system. The jaws, skull, and spine form a connected network – tension or restriction in one area affects the rest. Understanding those interrelationships allows me to guide patients toward the right practitioners and better results. Modern imaging like 3D CBCT scans further refines diagnosis, revealing airway, joint, and bone details with remarkable clarity. While some resist such innovation, meaningful progress always begins at the edges of convention.

Ultimately, collaboration matters more than competition. True professionals stay open-minded, learning from one another for the good of their patients. Criticism may come from those unwilling to look deeper, but ethical care means respect – for colleagues, evidence, and every child we help. Seeing young patients breathe easier, sleep better, and grow stronger is all the proof I need to keep learning, questioning, and evolving.

CHAPTER 23 KEY FINDINGS

- When children are given the right environment to grow, nature often exceeds expectations.
- Healing is a team effort – progress happens when practitioners and parents work together with openness and trust.
- The ultimate goal is independence: when healthy functions become second nature, growth and confidence can flourish on their own.

Parents: where do you go from here?

As a parent, you are the expert on your child. You know their moods, their rhythms, their quirks. And when something doesn't feel right, that inner voice deserves to be heard and trusted.

If you've noticed ongoing challenges in your child's development, such as difficulties with feeding, breathing, sleep, speech, learning, behavior, or physical discomfort, it's essential to consider that these may not be isolated problems. Instead, they could be signs of underlying functional health issues that are affecting your child's overall wellbeing and development.

Many of the signs – like mouth breathing, poor sleep, snoring, teeth grinding, a high palate, dark circles under the eyes, or even frequent tantrums – are often dismissed as 'normal' phases or just part of growing up. But these symptoms, especially when they persist or appear together, may point to a need for deeper investigation into how your child is functioning, not just how they appear on the surface.

What you can do

1. Start with observation

Begin by noting what you see and hear:

- How does your child breathe: through the mouth or nose?
- Is their mouth often open during the day or night?
- Do they snore, grind their teeth, or wake frequently?
- Are they picky eaters or struggling with textures or chewing?
- Do they seem constantly tired, distracted, or emotionally reactive?
- Are there signs of delayed speech or difficulty with sounds?

Keep a journal of these signs. Patterns are powerful tools when advocating for your child.

2. Seek the right support

No single professional will have all the answers, so consider a multidisciplinary approach. The right team might include:

- **Myofunctional dentist or orthodontist** – especially those trained in airway development, oral functions, and tethered oral tissues
- **Speech and language therapist** – for oral motor skills, feeding, speech
- **Orofacial myofunctional therapist** – for tongue posture, breathing, and oral habits
- **ENT specialist** – to evaluate tonsils, adenoids, sinus, and ear issues
- **Lactation consultant or feeding specialist** – for infants with feeding problems

- **Pediatric craniosacral or neurodevelopmental chiropractor or osteopath** (for structural imbalances, fascial restrictions, and neurological integration)
- **Pediatrician or integrative health practitioner** (to coordinate care and investigate root causes like allergies or sleep disorders).

Choose practitioners who take your concerns seriously and understand functional, rather than just structural, health. One of them can become the director of your child's health journey. A practitioner with a functional understanding tends to build a team around the patient to help them from a holistic approach.

3. Address root causes, not just symptoms

Rather than only managing behavior, academic performance, or sleep with surface-level fixes, focus on what might be driving these issues. For example:

- Mouth breathing and sleep disruption can reduce oxygen to the brain, impacting attention and behavior.
- A restricted tongue from a tongue tie can interfere with feeding, speech, breathing, and jaw development.
- Poor sleep and breathing can cause emotional volatility, learning difficulties, and even pain.

When you treat the cause - not just the outward expression - your child can begin to thrive.

4. Be patient, but proactive

Early intervention can change the trajectory of your child's development. However, even if your child is older, it's never too late. Functional health is adaptable, and the body can respond beautifully to the right support. Once you are on the journey, remember to allow and give time, because developing and establishing health takes time.

5. Trust your gut

You may be told 'they'll grow out of it' or 'it's just a phase'. While well-meaning, these responses can delay meaningful help. If something doesn't sit right with you, keep asking questions and seeking answers. You are your child's strongest advocate.

Final thoughts

Raising a child with functional health challenges can be overwhelming, but you are not alone. The signs your child is showing are not failures; they are **messages from the body** asking for help. And with the right support, many of these challenges can be addressed in ways that open up a future of greater ease, better health, and a child who feels more at home in their body and mind.

By recognizing the interconnectedness of feeding, breathing, sleeping, movement, and emotional regulation, you're already taking the first and most powerful step: seeing your child not in parts, but as a whole.

You don't need to have all the answers. But you do need to take the next step. And it begins with listening: to your child and to yourself.

Acknowledgements

This work is a reflection of not just my own efforts, but of the countless people whose love, guidance, and inspiration have carried me to this point. I could not have done this alone, and I wouldn't have wanted to.

First and foremost, thank you to Ethan, Sally, and your beautiful family for allowing me to share your journey. You are inspirational and fearless. Your strength and determination resonate deeply in countless hearts. We have all learned a great deal from you, as you set the example for many to follow.

To my wife. Your love has been my anchor and my light. Through every late night, every doubt, and every moment I questioned myself, you stood by me with unwavering strength and grace. Your sacrifices, often quiet and unseen, made all of this possible. This achievement is as much yours as it is mine.

To my children. You are my greatest motivation and my deepest source of joy. Your laughter, your questions, your hugs at the end of long days – these are the moments that remind me why I keep going. I hope, one day, this work inspires you as much as you inspire me.

To my mother, my father (who passed away when I was 14 years old), and my family. Thank you for standing by me, for shaping me, and for lifting me up through every phase of this journey.

Your support has been my foundation, and I carry your love with me in everything I do.

To my friends and peers. Thank you for your encouragement, your honesty, and your presence. Whether through shared struggles or shared celebrations, your companionship has made this journey richer and more meaningful.

To my teachers and mentors. Your wisdom and guidance shaped not just my thinking but who I am. Thank you for challenging me to grow, for holding me to high standards, and for always making space for my questions.

To my patients and their families. Thank you for your trust, your vulnerability, and your courage. You have taught me lessons that no textbook ever could. Your stories live within me and continue to shape my work.

To my team at The Myofunctional Centres. Thank you for your dedication, your skill, and your unwavering belief in our shared mission. This could not have been done without your hard work, your heart, and your tireless effort. You made the impossible feel possible.

To my book writing coach, my publisher, my editor, and everyone involved in creating this book. You are all amazing in your own individual ways. Thank you for making this process a joy, especially for a first-time author.

To the pioneers and trailblazers, those who test boundaries, break barriers, and boldly push the limits of possibility. Thank you for lighting the path. Your courage inspires us all to keep striving, questioning, and progressing.

And finally, to my dogs. Thank you for your unconditional love, for sitting beside me during long nights of writing, for reminding me to take breaks, and for being a quiet source of calm and joy. You have no idea how much you've helped, just by being there.

To each of you, thank you. This book is not mine alone. It belongs to all of us.

References

Al Ali, A, Richmond, S, Popat, H, et al. 'The influence of snoring, mouth breathing, and apnoea on facial morphology in late childhood: a three-dimensional study.' *BMJ Open* 2015;5:e009027. doi: 10.1136/bmjopen-2015-009027.

Al-Bitar, ZB, Al-Omari, IK, Sonbol, HN, Al-Ahmad, HT, and Cunningham, SJ. 'Bullying among Jordanian schoolchildren, its effects on school performance, and the contribution of general physical and dentofacial features.' *American Journal of Orthodontics and Dentofacial Orthopedics* 144, no. 6 (2013): 872-878.

Al-Hammad, Nouf S, Lujain A Hakeem, and Fouad S Salama. 'Oral health status of children with obstructive sleep apnea and snoring.' *Pediatric Dentistry* 37, no. 1 (2015): 35-39.

Alexopoulos, Emmanouel I, Eleni Kostadima, Ioanna Pagonari, Elias Zintzaras, Konstantinos Gourgoulianis, and Athanasios G Kaditis. 'Association between primary nocturnal enuresis and habitual snoring in children.' *Urology* 68, no. 2 (2006): 406-409.

Amat P, Tran Lu Y É. 'Apport de la rééducation myofonctionnelle orofaciale au traitement du syndrome d'apnées obstructives du sommeil : une revue systématique de la littérature [The contribution of orofacial myofunctional reeducation to the treatment of obstructive sleep apnoea syndrome (OSA): a systematic review of the literature].' *Orthod Fr.* 2019 Dec 1;90(3-4):343-370. French. doi: 10.1051/orthodfr/2019035. PMID: 34643521.

Avis, Kristin T, Karen L Gamble, and David C Schwebel. 'Obstructive sleep apnea syndrome increases pedestrian injury risk in children.' *The Journal of Pediatrics* 166, no. 1 (2015): 109-114.

Bahr, Diane. *Nobody Ever Told Me (or My Mother) That!: Everything from Bottles and Breathing to Healthy Speech Development.* Future Horizons, 2010.

Balasubramaniam, Ramesh, GD Klasser, PA Cistulli, and GJ Lavigne. 'The link between sleep bruxism, sleep disordered breathing, and temporomandibular disorders: an evidence-based review.' *J Dent Sleep Med* 1, no. 1 (2014): 27-37.

Ballard JL, Auer CE, Khoury JC. 'Ankyloglossia: assessment, incidence, and effect of frenuloplasty on the breastfeeding dyad.' *Pediatrics.* 2002 Nov;110(5):e63. doi: 10.1542/peds.110.5.e63. PMID: 12415069.

Bandyopadhyay, Anuja, Kellie Kaneshiro, Macario Camacho. 'Effect of myofunctional therapy on children with obstructive sleep apnea: a meta-analysis.' *Sleep Medicine*, 75 (2020): 210-217.

Barros, Juliana RC, Helena MG Becker, and Jorge A Pinto. 'Evaluation of atopy among mouth-breathing pediatric patients referred for treatment to a tertiary care center.' *Jornal de Pediatria* 82 (2006): 458-464.

Baxter R, Merkel-Walsh R, Lahey L, Knutsen C, Zaghi S. 'The buccal frenum: trends in diagnosis and indications for treatment of buccal ties among 466 healthcare professionals.' *J Oral Rehabil.* 2024 Feb;51(2):369-379. doi: 10.1111/joor.13609. Epub 2023 Oct 12. PMID: 37823364.

Baxter, Richard, and DMD Baxter. *Tongue-Tied: How a Tiny String Under the Tongue Impacts Nursing, Speech, Feeding, and More.* Alabama Tongue-Tie Center Inc., 2018.

Beebe, Dean W, and David Gozal. 'Obstructive sleep apnea and the prefrontal cortex: towards a comprehensive model linking nocturnal upper airway obstruction to daytime cognitive and behavioral deficits.' *Journal of Sleep Research* 11, no. 1 (2002): 1-16.

Beebe, Dean W, Joseph Rausch, Kelly C Byars, Bruce Lanphear, and Kimberly Yolton. 'Persistent snoring in preschool children: predictors and behavioral and developmental correlates.' *Pediatrics* 130, no. 3 (2012): 382-389.

Belmehdi A, Harti KE, Wady WE. 'Ankyloglossia as an oral functional problem and its surgical management.' *Dent Med Probl.* 2018 Apr-Jun;55(2):213-216. doi: 10.17219/dmp/85708. PMID: 30152627.

Benkert, Kimberly K. 'The effectiveness of orofacial myofunctional therapy in improving dental occlusion.' *The International Journal of Orofacial Myology:* 23 (1997): 35-46.

Berry J, Griffiths M, Westcott C. 'A double-blind, randomized, controlled trial of tongue-tie division and its immediate effect on breastfeeding.' *Breastfeed Med.* 2012 Jun;7(3):189-93. doi: 10.1089/bfm.2011.0030. Epub 2011 Oct 14. PMID: 21999476.

Berry, Janet, Mervyn Griffiths, and Carolyn Westcott. 'A double-blind, randomized, controlled trial of tongue-tie division and its immediate effect on breastfeeding.' *Breastfeeding Medicine* 7, no. 3 (2012): 189-193.

Bonuck K, Freeman K, Chervin RD, Xu L. 'Sleep-disordered breathing in a population-based cohort: behavioral outcomes at 4 and 7 years.' *Pediatrics.* 2012 Apr;129(4):e857-65. doi: 10.1542/peds.2011-1402. Epub 2012 Mar 5. PMID: 22392181; PMCID: PMC3313633.

Borovich, Adi, Yakov Sivan, Michal Greenfeld, and Riva Tauman. 'The history of primary snoring in children: the effect of adenotonsillectomy.' *Sleep Medicine* 17 (2016): 13-17.

Botzer E, Quinzi V, Salvati SE, Coceani Paskay L, Saccomanno S. 'Myofunctional therapy Part 3: Tongue function and breastfeeding as precursor of oronasal functions.' *Eur J Paediatr Dent.* 2021 Sep;22(3):248-250. doi: 10.23804/ejpd.2021.22.03.13. PMID: 34544256.

Bourjeily, Ghada, Valery A Danilack, Margaret H Bublitz, Janet Muri, Karen Rosene-Montella, and Heather Lipkind. 'Maternal obstructive sleep apnea and neonatal birth outcomes in a population-based sample.' *Sleep Medicine* 66 (2020): 233-240.

Boyd K, Saccomanno S, Lewis CJ, Coceani Paskay L, Quinzi V, Marzo G. 'Myofunctional therapy Part 1: Culture, industrialization, and the shrinking human face.' *Eur J Paediatr Dent.* 2021;22(1):80-81. doi: 10.23804/ejpd.2021.22.01.15. PMID: 33719489.

Boyd KL. 'A century of adenotonsillectomy's failure to fully resolve sleep-disordered breathing: mild malocclusions are maybe not so mild?' *J Clin Sleep Med.* 2020;16(8):1229-1230.

Boyd, Kevin L. 'Assessment and therapies for sleep and sleep-related breathing disorders associated with atopic disease in children: a dental perspective.' In *Allergy and Sleep: Basic Principles and Clinical Practice*, pp. 423-434. Cham: Springer International Publishing, 2019.

Boyd, Kevin L. 'Darwinian Dentistry.' *Journal of American Orthodontic Society* (2012): 28-33.

Buryk M, Bloom D, Shope T. 'Efficacy of neonatal release of ankyloglossia: a randomized trial.' *Pediatrics.* 2011 Aug;128(2):280-8. doi: 10.1542/peds.2011-0077. Epub 2011 Jul 18. PMID: 21768318.

Bussi MT, Corrêa CC, Cassettari AJ, Giacomin LT, Faria AC, Moreira APSM, Magalhães I, Cunha MOD, Weber SAT, Zancanella E, Machado Júnior AJ. 'Is ankyloglossia associated with obstructive sleep apnea?' *Braz J Otorhinolaryngol.* 2022 Nov-Dec;88 (Suppl 1):S156-S162. doi: 10.1016/j.bjorl.2021.09.008. Epub 2021 Nov 5. PMID: 34895868; PMCID: PMC9734261.

Camacho, Macario, Victor Certal, Jose Abdullatif, Soroush Zaghi, Chad M. Ruoff, Robson Capasso, and Clete A. Kushida. 'Myofunctional therapy to treat obstructive sleep apnea: a systematic review and meta-analysis.' *Sleep* 38, no. 5 (2015): 669-675.

Capdevila, Oscar Sans, Leila Kheirandish-Gozal, Ehab Dayyat, and David Gozal. 'Pediatric obstructive sleep apnea: complications, management, and long-term outcomes.' *Proceedings of the American Thoracic Society* 5, no. 2 (2008): 274-282.

Carrasco-Llatas, Marina, Carlos O'Connor-Reina, and Christian Calvo-Henriquez. 'The role of myofunctional therapy in treating sleep-disordered breathing: a state-of-the-art review.' *International Journal of Environmental Research and Public Health* 18, no. 14 (2021): 7291.

Carvalho, Fernando Rodrigues, Débora Aparecida Lentini-Oliveira, Graziele Maria Missiano Carvalho, Lucila Bizari Fernandes Prado, Gilmar Fernandes Prado, and Luciane Bizari Coin Carvalho. 'Sleep-disordered breathing and orthodontic variables in children – pilot study.'

International Journal of Pediatric Otorhinolaryngology 78, no. 11 (2014): 1965-1969.

Chen, Xiaoxian, Bin Xia, and Lihong Ge. 'Effects of breast-feeding duration, bottle-feeding duration, and non-nutritive sucking habits on the occlusal characteristics of primary dentition.' *BMC Pediatrics* 15, no. 1 (2015): 46.

Chervin, Ronald D, Kristen Hedger Archbold, James E Dillon, Parviz Panahi, Kenneth J Pituch, Ronald E Dahl, and Christian Guilleminault. 'Inattention, hyperactivity, and symptoms of sleep-disordered breathing.' *Pediatrics* 109, no. 3 (2002): 449-456.

Chmura L. 'Obstructive sleep apnea and the orthodontist.' *J Clin Orthod*. 2022 Jan;56(1):9-22. PMID: 35704887.

Cho A, Kelsberg G, Safranek S. 'Clinical inquiries. When should you treat tongue-tie in a newborn?' *J Fam Pract*. 2010 Dec;59(12):712a-b. PMID: 21135930.

Choi JY, Lee K. 'Effects of four first premolar extraction on the upper airway dimension in non-growing class I skeletal patients: a systematic review.' *J Oral Med Dent Res*. 3(1) (2022): 1-16.

Corrêa, Camila de Castro, and Giédre Berretin-Felix. 'Myofunctional therapy applied to upper airway resistance syndrome: a case report.' In *CoDAS*, vol. 27, pp. 604-609. Sociedade Brasileira de Fonoaudiologia, 2015.

Costa CTD, Shqair AQ, Azevedo MS, Goettems ML, Bonow MLM, Romano AR. 'Pacifier use modifies the association between breastfeeding and malocclusion: a cross-sectional study.' *Braz Oral Res*. 2018 Oct 11;32:e101. doi: 10.1590/1807-3107bor-2018.vol32.0101. PMID: 30328893.

D'Ascanio, Luca, Carla Lancione, Giorgio Pompa, Elena Rebuffini, Nicola Mansi, and Marco Manzini. 'Craniofacial growth in children with nasal septum deviation: a cephalometric comparative study.' *International Journal of Pediatric Otorhinolaryngology* 74, no. 10 (2010): 1180-1183.

Dao Anh Hoang, Van Nhat Thang Le, Tam Minh Nguyen, Triin Jagomägi. 'Orofacial dysfunction screening examinations in children with sleep-disordered breathing symptoms.' *Journal of Clinical Pediatric Dentistry*. 2023; 47(4): 25-34. doi: 10.22514/jocpd.2023.032.

Dezio, M, Piras, A, Gallottini, L, & Denotti, G. 'Tongue-tie, from embryology to treatment: a literature review.' *Journal of Pediatric and Neonatal Individualized Medicine (JPNIM)*, 4(1), e040101.

Dhadse PV, Patil RT, Salian SS, Oza RR, Punse SD. 'Laser-assisted lingual frenectomy: a case report.' *Cureus*. 2024 Apr 30;16(4):e59412. doi: 10.7759/cureus.59412. PMID: 38826594; PMCID: PMC11139779.

Durán-Cantolla, Joaquín, Mohammad Hamdan Alkhraisat, Cristina Martínez-Null, José Javier Aguirre, Elena Rubio Guinea, and Eduardo Anitua. 'Frequency of obstructive sleep apnea syndrome in dental patients with tooth wear.' *Journal of Clinical Sleep Medicine* 11, no. 4 (2015): 445-450.

Eastman, NJ. 'Mount Everest in utero.' *Am J Obstet Gynecol.* 1954 Apr;67(4):701-11. doi: 10.1016/0002-9378(54)90098-8. PMID: 13148241.

Edmunds, Janet, Miles, Sandra, and Fulbrook, Paul. 'Tongue-tie and breastfeeding: a review of the literature.' *Breastfeeding Review* 19: 19-26.

Enlow, Donald H, Mark G Hans, and Larry McGrew. *Essentials of Facial Growth*. Vol. 35. Philadelphia: Saunders, 1996.

Ezzat, WF, Samia A Fawaz, and Samar M Farid. 'Impact of sleep-disordered breathing and its treatment on children with primary nocturnal enuresis.' *Swiss Medical Weekly* 141, no. 2526 (2011): w13216-w13216.

Fensterseifer, Giovana Serrão, Oswaldo Carpes, Luc Louis Maurice Weckx, and Viviane Feller Martha. 'Mouth breathing in children with learning disorders.' *Brazilian Journal of Otorhinolaryngology* 79 (2013): 620-624.

Ferreira, Natália Maria Ribeiro, Jarbas Francisco Fernandes Dos Santos, Mateus Bertolini Fernandes dos Santos, and Leonardo Marchini. 'Sleep bruxism associated with obstructive sleep apnea syndrome in children.' *CRANIO®* 33, no. 4 (2015): 251-255.

Ferrés-Amat, E, Pastor-Vera, T, Ferrés-Amat, E, Mareque-Bueno, J, Prats-Armengol, J, and Ferrés-Padró, E. 'Multidisciplinary management of ankyloglossia in childhood: treatment of 101 cases. A protocol.' *Med Oral Patol Oral Cir Bucal*. 2016 Jan 1;21(1):e39-47.

Ferrés-Amat, E, Pastor-Vera, T, Rodriguez-Alessi, P, Ferrés-Amat, E, Mareque-Bueno, J, and Ferrés-Padró, E. 'The prevalence of ankyloglossia in 302 newborns with breastfeeding problems and sucking difficulties in Barcelona: a descriptive study.' *Eur J Paediatr Dent.* 2017 Dec;18(4):319-325. doi: 10.23804/ejpd.2017.18.04.10. PMID: 29380619.

Fidan, Tulin, and Vural Fidan. 'The impact of adenotonsillectomy on attention-deficit hyperactivity and disruptive behavioral symptoms.' *The Eurasian Journal of Medicine* 40, no. 1 (2008): 14.

Frosh, Adam, Carina Cruz, David Wellsted, and Joanna Stephens. 'Effect of a dairy diet on nasopharyngeal mucus secretion.' *The Laryngoscope* 129, no. 1 (2019): 13-17.

García-Righetti, G, and Islas-Tejera, A. 'Tongue-tie in babies: diagnosis and laser frenectomy. Case report.' *Journal of Oral Research* 11(1): 1-10.

Gelb, M, Montrose, J, Paglia, L, Saccomanno, S, Quinzi, V, and Marzo, G. 'Myofunctional therapy Part 2: Prevention of dentofacial disorders.' *Eur J Paediatr Dent.* 2021 Jun;22(2):163-167. doi: 10.23804/ejpd.2021.22.02.15. PMID: 34238010.

Ghaheri, Bobak A, Melissa Cole, Sarah C Fausel, Maria Chuop, and Jess C Mace. 'Breastfeeding improvement following tongue-tie and lip-tie release: a prospective cohort study.' *The Laryngoscope* 127, no. 5 (2017): 1217-1223.

Goodwin, James L, Kris L Kaemingk, Ralph F Fregosi, Gerald M Rosen, Wayne J Morgan, Terry Smith, and Stuart F Quan. 'Parasomnias and sleep-disordered breathing in Caucasian and Hispanic children: the Tucson Children's Assessment of Sleep Apnea Study.' *BMC Medicine* 2, no. 1 (2004): 14.

Gozal, David, and Leila Kheirandish-Gozal. 'Cardiovascular morbidity in obstructive sleep apnea: oxidative stress, inflammation, and much more.' *American Journal of Respiratory and Critical Care Medicine* 177, no. 4 (2008): 369-375.

Gozal, David, Leila Kheirandish-Gozal, Rakesh Bhattacharjee, and Karen Spruyt. 'Neurocognitive and endothelial dysfunction in children with obstructive sleep apnea.' *Pediatrics* 126, no. 5 (2010): e1161-e1167.

Gozal, David. 'Obstructive sleep apnea in children: implications for the developing central nervous system.' In *Seminars in Pediatric Neurology*, vol. 15, no. 2, pp. 100-106. WB Saunders, 2008.

Gozal, David. 'Sleep-disordered breathing and school performance in children.' *Pediatrics* 102, no. 3 (1998): 616-620.

Grabowski, Rosemarie, Franka Stahl, Manja Gaebel, and Günther Kundt. 'Relationship between occlusal findings and orofacial myo-functional status in primary and mixed dentition: Part I: prevalence of malocclusions.' *Journal of Orofacial Orthopedics/Fortschritte der Kieferorthopädie* 68, no. 1 (2007): 26-37.

Grabowski, Rosemarie, Günther Kundt, and Franka Stahl. 'Interrelation between occlusal findings and orofacial myofunctional status in primary and mixed dentition: Part III: Interrelation between malocclusions and orofacial dysfunctions.' *Journal of Orofacial Orthopedics/Fortschritte der Kieferorthopädie* 68, no. 6 (2007): 462-476.

Graham, Tess. *Relief from Snoring and Sleep Apnea: A Step-by-Step Guide to Restful Sleep and Better Health Through Changing the Way You Breathe.* Createspace Independent Publishing Platform, 2014.

Guilleminault, C, Huseni, S, and Lo, L. 'A frequent phenotype for pediatric sleep apnoea: short lingual frenulum.' *ERJ Open Research* 2, no. 3 (2016): 00043-2016. doi: 10.1183/23120541.00043-2016. PMID: 27730205; PMCID: PMC5034598.

Guilleminault, Christian, and Kasey K Li. 'Maxillomandibular expansion for the treatment of sleep-disordered breathing: preliminary result.' *The Laryngoscope* 114, no. 5 (2004): 893-896.

Guilleminault, Christian, and Shannon S Sullivan. 'Towards restoration of continuous nasal breathing as the ultimate treatment goal in pediatric obstructive sleep apnea.' *Enliven: Pediatr Neonatol Biol* 1, no. 1 (2014): 001.

Guilleminault, Christian, and Vivien C Abad. 'Obstructive sleep apnea syndromes.' *Medical Clinics* 88, no. 3 (2004): 611-630.

Guilleminault, Christian, Ara Tilkian, and William C Dement. 'The sleep apnea syndromes.' *Annual Review of Medicine* (1976).

Guilleminault, Christian, Luciana Palombini, Rafael Pelayo, and Ronald D Chervin. 'Sleepwalking and sleep terrors in prepubertal children: what triggers them?' *Pediatrics* 111, no. 1 (2003): e17-e25.

Guilleminault, Christian, Rafael Pelayo, Damien Leger, Alex Clerk, and Robert CZ Bocian. 'Recognition of sleep-disordered breathing in children.' *Pediatrics* 98, no. 5 (1996): 871-882.

Guilleminault, Christian, Shannon S Sullivan, and Yu-shu Huang. 'Sleep-disordered breathing, orofacial growth, and prevention of obstructive sleep apnea.' *Sleep Medicine Clinics* 14, no. 1 (2019): 13-20.

Guilleminault, Christian, Vivien C Abad, Hsiao-Yean Chiu, Brandon Peters, and Stacey Quo. 'Missing teeth and pediatric obstructive sleep apnea.' *Sleep and Breathing* 20, no. 2 (2016): 561-568.

Guimarães, Kátia C, Luciano F Drager, Pedro R Genta, Bianca F Marcondes, and Geraldo Lorenzi-Filho. 'Effects of oropharyngeal exercises on patients with moderate obstructive sleep apnea syndrome.' *American Journal of Respiratory and Critical Care Medicine* 179, no. 10 (2009): 962-966.

Hakim, Fahed, Leila Kheirandish-Gozal, and David Gozal. 'Obesity and altered sleep: a pathway to metabolic derangements in children?' *Seminars in Pediatric Neurology*, vol. 22, no. 2, pp. 77-85. WB Saunders, 2015.

Hill, Catherine M, Alexandra M Hogan, Nwanneka Onugha, Dawn Harrison, Sara Cooper, Victoria J McGrigor, Avijit Datta, and Fenella J Kirkham. 'Increased cerebral blood flow velocity in children with mild sleep-disordered breathing: a possible association with abnormal neuropsychological function.' *Pediatrics* 118, no. 4 (2006): e1100-e1108.

Hill, RR, Lee, CS, and Pados, BF. 'The prevalence of ankyloglossia in children aged <1 year: a systematic review and meta-analysis.' *Pediatr Res.* 2021 Aug;90(2):259-266. doi: 10.1038/s41390-020-01239-y. Epub 2020 Nov 13. PMID: 33188284.

Hogan, Monica, Carolyn Westcott, and Mervyn Griffiths. 'Randomized, controlled trial of division of tongue-tie in infants with feeding problems.' *Journal of Paediatrics and Child Health* 41, no. 5-6 (2005): 246-250.

Huang, Boyen, Carla Lejarraga, Christopher S Franco, Yunlong Kang, Andrew Lee, John Abbott, Katsu Takahashi, Kazuhisa Bessho, and

Pongthorn Pumtang-On. 'Influence of non-orthodontic intervention on digit sucking and consequent anterior open bite: a preliminary study.' *International Dental Journal* 65, no. 5 (2015): 235-241.

Huang, Yu-Shu, Shih-Chieh Hsu, Christian Guilleminault, and Li-Chuan Chuang. 'Myofunctional therapy: role in pediatric OSA.' *Sleep Medicine Clinics* 14, no. 1 (2018): 135-142.

Huang, Yu-Shu, Stacey Quo, J Andrew Berkowski, and Christian Guilleminault. 'Short lingual frenulum and obstructive sleep apnea in children.' *Int J Pediatr Res* 1, no. 1 (2015): 273.

Hultcrantz, Elisabeth, and B Löfstrand Tideström. 'The development of sleep-disordered breathing from 4 to 12 years and dental arch morphology.' *International Journal of Pediatric Otorhinolaryngology* 73, no. 9 (2009): 1234-1241.

Iftikhar, Imran H, Christopher E Kline, and Shawn D Youngstedt. 'Effects of exercise training on sleep apnea: a meta-analysis.' *Lung* 192, no. 1 (2014): 175-184.

Ishii, Lisa, Chris Roxbury, Andres Godoy, Stacey Ishman, and Masaru Ishii. 'Does nasal surgery improve OSA in patients with nasal obstruction and OSA? A meta-analysis.' *Otolaryngology–Head and Neck Surgery* 153, no. 3 (2015): 326-333.

Jahn, Christoph, Haralampos Gouveris, and Christoph Matthias. 'Systemic inflammation in patients with compromised upper airway anatomy and primary snoring or mild obstructive sleep apnea.' *European Archives of Oto-Rhino-Laryngology* 273, no. 10 (2016): 3429-3433.

Jamieson, Andrew, Christian Guilleminault, Markku Partinen, and Maria Antonia Quera-Salva. 'Obstructive sleep apneic patients have craniomandibular abnormalities.' *Sleep* 9, no. 4 (1986): 469-477.

Jefferson, Yosh. 'Mouth breathing: adverse effects on facial growth, health, academics, and behavior.' *Gen Dent* 58, no. 1 (2010): 18-25.

Kato, Takafumi, Akira Mikami, Hideko Sugita, Hisae Muraki, Mutsumi Okura, Motoharu Ohi, and Mitsutaka Taniguchi. 'Negative association between self-reported jaw symptoms and apnea–hypopnea index in patients with symptoms of obstructive sleep apnea syndrome: a pilot study.' *Sleep and Breathing* 17, no. 1 (2013): 373-379.

Kayamori, Fabiane, and Esther Mandelbaum Gonçalves Bianchini. 'Effects of orofacial myofunctional therapy on the symptoms and physiological parameters of sleep breathing disorders in adults: a systematic review.' *Revista CEFAC* 19, no. 6 (2017): 868-878.

Keating, Genevieve M. 'Parent reports of chiropractic care for children: a preliminary report from 22,043 parents in Australia.' *J Clin Chiropr Pediatr* 20, no. 1 (2021): 1731-1732.

Keating, Genevieve, Cheryl Hawk, Lyndon Amorin-Woods, Deisy Amorin-Woods, Sharon Vallone, Ronald Farabaugh, Angela Todd et al. 'Clinical practice guideline for best practice management of pediatric patients by chiropractors: results of a Delphi consensus process.' *Journal of Integrative and Complementary Medicine* 30, no. 3 (2024): 216-232.

Kim, Jee Hyun, and Christian Guilleminault. 'The nasomaxillary complex, the mandible, and sleep-disordered breathing.' *Sleep and Breathing* 15, no. 2 (2011): 185-193.

Kim, Su-Jung, and Ki Beom Kim, eds. 'Orthodontics in obstructive sleep apnea patients: a guide to diagnosis, treatment planning, and interventions.' *Springer Nature*, 2019.

Klasser, Gary D, Nathalie Rei, and Gilles J Lavigne. 'Sleep bruxism etiology: the evolution of a changing paradigm.' *Journal of the Canadian Dental Association* (2015).

Kotlow, L. 'Lasers and soft tissue treatments for the pediatric dental patient.' *Alpha Omegan* 101, no. 3 (2008): 140-151. doi: 10.1016/j.aodf.2008.07.026. PMID: 19127931.

Kotlow, LA. 'The influence of the maxillary frenum on the development and pattern of dental caries on anterior teeth in breastfeeding infants: prevention, diagnosis, and treatment.' *Journal of Human Lactation* 26, no. 3 (2010): 304-308. doi: 10.1177/0890334410362520.

Kotlow, Larry. *SOS 4 TOTS*. The Troy Book Makers, 2016.

Kotlow, Lawrence. 'Infant gastroesophageal reflux (GER – benign infant acid reflux) or just plain aerophagia.' *International Journal of Child Health and Nutrition* 5, no. 1 (2016): 10-16.

Kotlow, Lawrence. 'Infant reflux and aerophagia associated with the maxillary lip-tie and ankyloglossia (tongue-tie).' *Clinical Lactation* 2 (2011): 25-29. doi: 10.1891/215805311807011467.

Lavigne, Gilles, Barry J Sessle, Manon Choinière, and Peter Soja. *Sleep and pain*. Lippincott Williams & Wilkins, 2015.

Lee, Chang Ho, Young Ju Kim, Sun Bin Lee, Chan Kee Yoo, and Hyoung-Mi Kim. 'Psychological screening for children with habitual snoring.' *International Journal of Pediatric Otorhinolaryngology* 78, no. 12 (2014): 2145-2150.

Lim, Shereen. *Breathe, Sleep, Thrive: Discover How Airway Health Can Unlock Your Child's Greater Health, Learning, and Potential*. Sparkle Publishing, 2022.

Lin, Steven. *The dental diet: the surprising link between your teeth, real food, and life-changing natural health*. Hay House, 2018.

Lyu, J, Ye, X, Chen, Y, Xia, Y, Zhu, J, Tong, S, Yin, Y, Qu, J, Li, S. 'Children's sleep may depend on maternal sleep duration during pregnancy: a retrospective study.' *Nat Sci Sleep* 12 (2020): 197-207. doi: 10.2147/NSS.S239001. PMID: 32210651; PMCID: PMC7071877.

Lyu, J, Xiuxia Ye, Yiting Chen, Yuanqing Xia, Jianzhen Zhu, Shilu Tong, Yong Yin, Jiajie Qu & Shenghui Li (2020) 'Children's sleep may depend on maternal sleep duration during pregnancy: a retrospective study,' *Nature and Science of Sleep*, 12, 197-207, DOI: 10.2147/NSS.S239001.

Macaluso, M, and D Hockenbury. 'Lingual, labial frenums: early detection can prevent health effects associated with tongue-tie.' Available at: rdhmag.com/articles/print 35 (2015).

Mahony, Derek, Agneta Karsten, and Sten Linder-Aronson. 'Effects of adenoidectomy and changed mode of breathing on incisor and molar dentoalveolar heights and anterior face heights.' *Australian Orthodontic Journal* 20, no. 2 (2004): 93-98.

Mahony, Derek, Niroj Bhattarai, Cascella Simona, Bucci Rosaria, Peter Borbély, Peter Petocz, Audrey Yoon, and Krisztina Kárpáti. 'Facial patterns and obstructive sleep apnea in children seeking orthodontic treatment: data from 3671 polysomnographic recordings.' *Orthodontics & Craniofacial Research* (2025).

Mahony, Derek. 'Refining occlusion with muscle balance to enhance long-term orthodontic stability.' *Malaysian Dental Journal* 31, no. 1 (2010).

Major, MP, H El-Hakim, M Witmans, PW Major, and C Flores-Mir. 'Adenoid hypertrophy in pediatric sleep-disordered breathing and craniofacial growth: the emerging role of dentistry.' *J Dent Sleep Med* 1, no. 2 (2014): 83-87.

Mandrawa, Donny, Mary Bourke, and Ignatius Bourke. 'A myofunctional chewing device as an early intervention tool for a child with achondroplasia and obstructive sleep apnea.' *International Journal of Orofacial Myology and Myofunctional Therapy* 50, no. 1 (2024): 1-8.

Marcus, Carole L, Lee J Brooks, Sally Davidson Ward, Kari A Draper, David Gozal, Ann C Halbower, Jacqueline Jones et al. 'Diagnosis and management of childhood obstructive sleep apnea syndrome.' *Pediatrics* 130, no. 3 (2012): e714-e755.

Marcus, Carole L, Reneé H Moore, Carol L Rosen, Bruno Giordani, Susan L Garetz, H Gerry Taylor, Ron B Mitchell et al. 'A randomized trial of adenotonsillectomy for childhood sleep apnea.' *New England Journal of Medicine* 368, no. 25 (2013): 2366-2376.

Martinot, Jean-Benoît, Frédéric Senny, Stéphane Denison, Valérie Cuthbert, Emmanuelle Gueulette, Hervé Guénard, and Jean-Louis Pépin. 'Mandibular movements identify respiratory effort in pediatric obstructive sleep apnea.' *Journal of Clinical Sleep Medicine* 11, no. 5 (2015): 567-574.

Matsuo, Koichiro, and Jeffrey B Palmer. 'Anatomy and physiology of feeding and swallowing: normal and abnormal.' *Clinics in Integrated Care* 16 (2023): 100139.

Mattoo, Khurshid, Brar, Anchal, and Kamarthi, Nagaraju. 'Psychosocial factors associated with ankyloglossia – a clinical case report.' *Journal of Medical Science and Clinical Research* 2 (2014): 2165-2169.

McKeown, Patrick G, and Manish Shah. *Close Your Mouth*. Buteyko Books, 2012.

McKeown, Patrick, and Martha Macaluso. 'Mouth breathing: physical, mental, and emotional consequences.' *Oral Health* 1 (2017).

McKeown, Patrick, Carlos O'Connor-Reina, and Guillermo Plaza. 'Breathing re-education and phenotypes of sleep apnea: a review.' *Journal of Clinical Medicine* 10, no. 3 (2021): 471.

McKeown, Patrick. *The Oxygen Advantage: Simple, Scientifically Proven Breathing Techniques*. William Morrow Paperbacks, 2015.

Messner, AH, and Lalakea, ML. 'The effect of ankyloglossia on speech in children.' *Otolaryngology Head and Neck Surgery* 127, no. 6 (2002): 539-545. doi: 10.1067/mhn.2002.129731. PMID: 12501105.

Mew, John RC. 'The postural basis of malocclusion: a philosophical overview.' *American Journal of Orthodontics and Dentofacial Orthopedics* 126, no. 6 (2004): 729-738.

Mew, John. 'Bioblock therapy.' *American Journal of Orthodontics* 76, no. 1 (1979): 29-50.

Mew, John. 'Facial changes in identical twins treated by different orthodontic techniques.' *World Journal of Orthodontics* 8, no. 2 (2007).

Mew, John. 'The influence of the tongue on dentofacial growth.' *The Angle Orthodontist* 85, no. 4 (2015): 715-715.

Mew, John. 'Tongue posture.' *British Journal of Orthodontics* 8, no. 4 (1981): 203-211.

Michaëlsson, Karl, Alicja Wolk, Sophie Langenskiöld, Samar Basu, Eva Warensjö Lemming, Håkan Melhus, and Liisa Byberg. 'Milk intake and risk of mortality and fractures in women and men: cohort studies.' *BMJ* 349 (2014).

Mills, N, Geddes, DT, Amirapu, S, and Mirjalili, SA. 'Understanding the lingual frenulum: histological structure, tissue composition, and implications for tongue tie surgery.' *International Journal of Otolaryngology* (2020): 1820978. doi: 10.1155/2020/1820978. PMID: 32774383; PMCID: PMC7391099.

Mills, N, Pransky, SM, Geddes, DT, and Mirjalili, SA. 'What is a tongue tie? Defining the anatomy of the in-situ lingual frenulum.' *Clinical Anatomy* 32, no. 6 (2019): 749-761. doi: 10.1002/ca.23343. Epub 2019 Feb 19. PMID: 30701608; PMCID: PMC6850428.

Moeller, Joy Lea, MP Macaluso, and Ruth Marsiliani. 'Treatment of myofunctional pathology.' *Sleep Disorders in Pediatric Dentistry* (2019): n. pag.

Moimaz, Suzely Adas Saliba, Artênio José Ísper Garbin, Arinilson Moreira Chaves Lima, Luiz Fernando Lolli, Orlando Saliba, and Cléa Adas Adas Saliba Garbin. 'Longitudinal study of habits leading to malocclusion development in childhood.' *BMC Oral Health* 14, no. 1 (2014): 96.

Moore, Sharon. *Sleep Wrecked Kids: Helping Parents Raise Happy, Healthy Kids, One Sleep at a Time*. Morgan James Publishing, 2019.

Moreno-Indias, Isabel, Marta Torres, Josep M Montserrat, Lidia Sanchez-Alcoholado, Fernando Cardona, Francisco J Tinahones, David Gozal et al. 'Intermittent hypoxia alters gut microbiota diversity in a mouse model of sleep apnea.' *European Respiratory Journal* 45, no. 4 (2015): 1055-1065.

Moschik, Christoph E, Margit Pichelmayer, Sandra Coulson, and Brigitte Wendl. 'Influence of myofunctional therapy on upper intercanine distance.' *J Dent Oral Disord Ther* 3, no. 1 (2015): 1-7.

Nestor, James. *Breath: Improve Your Health and Wellbeing by Discovering the Lost Art of Breathing*. Penguin UK, 2020.

Nihi, Valdeane Simone Cenci, Sandra Mara Maciel, Marta Essuane Jarrus, Fabio Mitugui Nihi, Carlos Luiz Fernando de Salles, Renata Correa Pascotto, and Mitsue Fujimaki. 'Pacifier-sucking habit duration and frequency on occlusal and myofunctional alterations in preschool children.' *Brazilian Oral Research* 29 (2014): 00-00.

O'Connor, Anahad. 'How the Sugar Industry Shifted Blame to Fat.' *New York Times* 12 (2016).

Oh, James S, Soroush Zaghi, Nora Ghodousi, Cynthia Peterson, Daniela Silva, Gilles J Lavigne, Audrey J Yoon. 'Determinants of probable sleep bruxism in a pediatric mixed dentition population: a multivariate analysis of mouth vs. nasal breathing, tongue mobility, and tonsil size.' *Sleep Medicine*, Volume 77, 2021, 7-13.

Oh, JS, Zaghi, S, Peterson, C, Law, CS, Silva, D, Yoon, AJ. 'Determinants of sleep-disordered breathing during the mixed dentition: development of a functional airway evaluation screening tool (FAIREST-6).' *Pediatr Dent.* 2021 Jul 15;43(4):262-272. PMID: 34467840.

Oishi, Shuji, Yasuhiro Shimizu, Jun Hosomichi, Yoichiro Kuma, Hisashi Nagai, Hideyuki Maeda, Risa Usumi-Fujita, et al. 'Intermittent Hypoxia Induces Disturbances in Craniofacial Growth and Defects in Craniofacial Morphology.' *Archives of Oral Biology* 61 (2016): 115-124.

Okeson, Jeffrey P. *Management of Temporomandibular Disorders and Occlusion*. St. Louis, MO: Elsevier/Mosby, 2013.

Oliveira, Marcelo Tomás de, Sandra Teixeira Bittencourt, Karina Marcon, Samia Destro, and Jefferson Ricardo Pereira. 'Sleep bruxism and anxiety level in children.' *Brazilian Oral Research* 29 (2015): 1-5.

Olivi, G, A Signore, M Olivi, and MD Genovese. 'Lingual frenectomy: functional evaluation and new therapeutical approach.' *Eur J Paediatr Dent* 13, no. 2 (2012): 101-106.

Olivi, Giovanni, Fred S Margolis, and Maria Daniela Genovese. *Pediatric Laser Dentistry: A User's Guide*. Quintessence Pub Co, 2011.

Page, David C, and Derek Mahony. 'The airway, breathing and orthodontics.' *Todays FDA* 22, no. 2 (2010): 43-47.

Parisi, Pasquale, Nicoletta Pietropaoli, Alessandro Ferretti, Raffaella Nenna, Gerarda Mastrogiorgio, M Del Pozzo, Luigi Principessa, Margherita Bonamico, and MP Villa. 'Role of the gluten-free diet on neurological-EEG findings and sleep disordered breathing in children with celiac disease.' *Seizure* 25 (2015): 181-183.

Park, Sungchan, Jung Min Lee, Chang Sun Sim, Jae Gi Kim, Jung Gwon Nam, Tae-Hoon Lee, Myung Woul Han, Joong Keun Kwon, and Jong Cheol Lee. 'Impact of adenotonsillectomy on nocturnal enuresis in children with sleep-disordered breathing: a prospective study.' *The Laryngoscope* 126, no. 5 (2016): 1241-1245.

Paruthi, Shalini, Carol L Rosen, Rui Wang, Jia Weng, Carole L Marcus, Ronald D Chervin, Jeffrey J Stanley, Eliot S Katz, Raouf Amin, and Susan Redline. 'End-tidal carbon dioxide measurement during pediatric polysomnography: signal quality, association with apnea severity, and prediction of neurobehavioral outcomes.' *Sleep* 38, no. 11 (2015): 1719-1726.

Peres, KG, Cascaes, AM, Peres, MA, Demarco, FF, Santos, IS, Matijasevich, A, Barros, AJ. 'Exclusive breastfeeding and risk of dental malocclusion.' *Pediatrics.* 2015 Jul;136(1):e60-67. doi: 10.1542/peds.2014-3276. Epub 2015 Jun 15. PMID: 26077480.

Poachanukoon, Orapan, and Maleewan Kitcharoensakkul. 'Snoring and sleep problems in children with and without allergic rhinitis: a case control study.' *J Med Assoc Thai* 98, no. Suppl 2 (2015): S138-144.

Porges, Stephen W. 'Polyvagal theory: a science of safety.' *Frontiers in Integrative Neuroscience* 16 (2022): 871227.

Porges, Stephen W. 'The polyvagal perspective.' *Biological Psychology* 74, no. 2 (2007): 116-143.

Porges, Stephen W. 'The polyvagal theory: new insights into adaptive reactions of the autonomic nervous system.' *Cleveland Clinic Journal of Medicine* 76, no. Suppl 2 (2009): S86.

Porges, Stephen W. 'The polyvagal theory: phylogenetic contributions to social behavior.' *Physiology & Behavior* 79, no. 3 (2003): 503-513.

Pradhan, Suchetan, Effath Yasmin, and Amrita Mehta. 'Management of posterior ankyloglossia using the Er,Cr:YSGG laser.' *International Journal of Laser Dentistry* 2 (2012): 41-46. 10.5005/jp-journals-10022-1016.

Price, Weston A, and Trung Nguyen. *Nutrition and Physical Degeneration: A Comparison of Primitive and Modern Diets and Their Effects.* EnCognitive.com, 2016.

Rabasco, Jole, Alessandro Vigo, Ottavio Vitelli, Silvia Noce, Nicoletta Pietropaoli, Melania Evangelisti, and Maria Pia Villa. 'Apparent life-threatening events could be a wake-up call for sleep disordered breathing.' *Pediatric Pulmonology* 51, no. 12 (2016): 1403-1408.

Ramirez-Yañez, German, Anatans Sidlauskas, E Junior, and J Fluter. 'Dimensional changes in dental arches after treatment with a prefabricated functional appliance.' *Journal of Clinical Pediatric Dentistry* 31, no. 4 (2007): 279-283.

Ramirez-Yañez, German, and Paulo Faria. 'Early treatment of a class II, division 2 malocclusion with the trainer for kids (T4K): a case report.' *Journal of Clinical Pediatric Dentistry* 32, no. 4 (2008): 325-329.

Restrepo, Claudia Cecilia, Marcela Tirado, and Kelly Juliette Jimenez. 'Association of sleep bruxism and dental plaque factors on signs of periodontal disease in children in the mixed dentition.' *International Journal of Paediatric Dentistry* 26, no. 6 (2016): 477-485.

Ribeiro, GC, Dos Santos, ID, Santos, AC, Paranhos, LR, César, CP. 'Influence of the breathing pattern on the learning process: a systematic review of literature.' *Braz J Otorhinolaryngol.* 2016 Jul-Aug;82(4):466-478. doi: 10.1016/j.bjorl.2015.08.026. Epub 2016 Jan 7. PMID: 26832637; PMCID: PMC9448999.

Ricordi, C, Garcia-Contreras, M, and Farnetti, S. 'Diet and inflammation: possible effects on immunity, chronic diseases, and life span.' *Journal of the American College of Nutrition* 34 (2015): 10–13.

Roberts, Soleil D, Hitesh Kapadia, Geoff Greenlee, and Maida L Chen. 'Midfacial and dental changes associated with nasal positive airway pressure in children with obstructive sleep apnea and craniofacial conditions.' *Journal of Clinical Sleep Medicine* 12, no. 4 (2016): 469-475.

Rosen, Carol L, Rui Wang, H Gerry Taylor, Carole L Marcus, Eliot S Katz, Shalini Paruthi, Raanan Arens, et al. 'Utility of symptoms to predict treatment outcomes in obstructive sleep apnea syndrome.' *Pediatrics* 135, no. 3 (2015): e662-e671.

Ruoff, Chad M, and Christian Guilleminault. 'Orthodontics and sleep-disordered breathing.' *Sleep and Breathing* 16, no. 2 (2012): 271-273.

Sahin, Unal, Onder Ozturk, Mustafa Ozturk, Necla Songur, Ahmet Bircan, and Ahmet Akkaya. 'Habitual snoring in primary school children: prevalence and association with sleep-related disorders and school performance.' *Medical Principles and Practice* 18, no. 6 (2009): 458-465.

Sanders, Anne E, Aderonke A Akinkugbe, Gary D Slade, and Greg K Essick. 'Tooth loss and obstructive sleep apnea signs and symptoms in the U.S. population.' *Sleep and Breathing* 20, no. 3 (2016): 1095-1102.

Seehra, J, Fleming, PS, Newton, T, DiBiase, AT. 'Bullying in orthodontic patients and its relationship to malocclusion, self-esteem and oral health-related quality of life.' *J Orthod.* 2011 Dec;38(4):247-256.

Seemann, Jana, Günther Kundt, and Franka Stahl de Castrillon. 'Relationship between occlusal findings and orofacial myofunctional status in primary and mixed dentition: Part IV: interrelation between space conditions and orofacial dysfunctions.' *Journal of Orofacial Orthopedics/Fortschritte der Kieferorthopädie* 72, no. 1 (2011): 21-32.

Sekizuka, Hiromitsu, Naohiko Osada, and Yoshihiro J Akashi. 'Effect of oral appliance therapy on blood pressure in Japanese patients with obstructive sleep apnea.' *Clinical and Experimental Hypertension* 38, no. 4 (2016): 404-408.

Shapiro, Peter A. 'Effects of nasal obstruction on facial development.' *Journal of Allergy and Clinical Immunology* 81, no. 5 (1988): 967-971.

Šidlauskienė, Monika, Dalia Smailienė, Kristina Lopatienė, Emilis Čekanauskas, Rūta Pribuišienė, and Mantas Šidlauskas. 'Relationships between malocclusion, body posture, and nasopharyngeal pathology in pre-orthodontic children.' *Medical Science Monitor: International Medical Journal of Experimental and Clinical Research* 21 (2015): 1765.

Siegel, S. 'Aerophagia induced reflux in breastfeeding infants with ankyloglossia and shortened maxillary labial frenula (tongue and lip tie).' *International Journal of Clinical Pediatrics* 5, no. 1 (2016): 6-8.

Slagter, KW, Raghoebar, GM, Hamming, I, Meijer, J, Vissink, A. 'Effect of frenotomy on breastfeeding and reflux: results from the BRIEF prospective longitudinal cohort study.' *Clin Oral Investig.* 2021 Jun;25(6):3431-3439. doi: 10.1007/s00784-020-03665-y. Epub 2020 Dec 14. PMID: 33315177; PMCID: PMC8137608.

Srinivasan, Bhadrinath, and Arun B Chitharanjan. 'Skeletal and dental characteristics in subjects with ankyloglossia.' *Progress in Orthodontics* 14, no. 1 (2013): 44.

Stahl, Franka, Rosemarie Grabowski, Manja Gaebel, and Günther Kundt. 'Relationship between occlusal findings and orofacial myofunctional status in primary and mixed dentition: Part II: prevalence of orofacial dysfunctions.' *Journal of Orofacial Orthopedics/Fortschritte der Kieferorthopädie* 68, no. 2 (2007): 74-90.

Sum, FH, Zhang, L, Ling, HT, Yeung, CP, Li, KY, Wong, HM, Yang, Y. 'Association of breastfeeding and three-dimensional dental arch relationships in primary dentition.' *BMC Oral Health.* 2015 Mar 10;15:30. doi:10.1186/s12903-015-0010-1. PMID:25886754; PMCID: PMC4358868.

Suzuki, Masaaki, Taiji Furukawa, Akira Sugimoto, Koji Katada, Ryosuke Kotani, and Takayuki Yoshizawa. 'Relationship between oral flow patterns, nasal obstruction, and respiratory events during sleep.' *Journal of Clinical Sleep Medicine* 11, no. 8 (2015): 855-860.

Tan, Hui-Leng, David Gozal, and Leila Kheirandish-Gozal. 'Obstructive sleep apnea in children: a critical update.' *Nature and Science of Sleep* (2013): 109-123.

Tanya, Dr, Lele, Priya, and Patil, Dr 'Ankyloglossia: treatment with surgical lasers – a case report.' *IOSR Journal of Dental and Medical Sciences* 13 (2014): 61-64. doi: 10.9790/0853-13726164.

Turzo, Tasha. 'The ALF approach.' *CRANIO®* 37, no. 2 (2019): 72-73.

van den Heuvel, MI, Hect, JL, Smarr, BL, Qawasmeh, T, Kriegsfeld, LJ, Barcelona, J, Hijazi, KE, and Thomason, ME. 'Maternal stress during pregnancy alters fetal cortico-cerebellar connectivity in utero and increases child sleep problems after birth.' *Sci Rep* 11, no. 1 (2021): 2228. doi: 10.1038/s41598-021-81681-y. PMID: 33500446; PMCID: PMC7838320.

Van Dyck, Claire, Aline Dekeyser, Elien Vantricht, Eric Manders, Ann Goeleven, Steffen Fieuws, and Guy Willems. 'The effect of orofacial myofunctional treatment in children with anterior open bite and tongue dysfunction: a pilot study.' *European Journal of Orthodontics* 38, no. 3 (2016): 227-234.

Vaz, Anna Cecilia, and Pavithra M Bai. 'Lingual frenulum and malocclusion: an overlooked tissue or a minor issue.' *Indian Journal of Dental Research* 26, no. 5 (2015): 488-492.

Verbeke, J, Meerschman, I, Dhondt, K, De Leenheer, E, Willekens, J, Van Lierde, K, and Claeys, S. 'Orofacial myofunctional therapy: investigating a novel therapeutic approach for pediatric obstructive sleep apnea in children with and without down syndrome – a study protocol.' *Children (Basel)* 12, no. 6 (2025): 737. doi: 10.3390/children12060737. PMID: 40564695; PMCID: PMC12191010.

Verma, Roshan K, Jai Richo Johnson, Manoj Goyal, N Banumathy, Upendra Goswami, and Naresh K Panda. 'Oropharyngeal exercises in the treatment of obstructive sleep apnea: our experience.' *Sleep and Breathing* 20, no. 4 (2016): 1193-1201.

Villa, Maria Pia, Melania Evangelisti, Susy Martella, Mario Barreto, and Marco Del Pozzo. 'Can myofunctional therapy increase tongue tone and reduce symptoms in children with sleep-disordered breathing?' *Sleep and Breathing* 21, no. 4 (2017): 1025-1032.

Vinha, Pedro, and Mello-Filho, Francisco. 'Evidence of a preventive effect of breastfeeding on obstructive sleep apnea in children and adults.' *Journal of Human Lactation* 33 (2017): 089033441668200. doi: 10.1177/0890334416682006.

Weitzberg, Eddie, and Jon ON Lundberg. 'Humming greatly increases nasal nitric oxide.' *American Journal of Respiratory and Critical Care Medicine* 166, no. 2 (2002): 144-145.

William, Kevin, and Derek Mahony. 'The effects of enlarged adenoids on a developing malocclusion.' *Journal of Pediatric Dental Care* 13, no. 3 (2007).

Yoon, A, Zaghi, S, Weitzman, R, Ha, S, Law, CS, Guilleminault, C, and Liu, SYC. 'Toward a functional definition of ankyloglossia: validating current grading scales for lingual frenulum length and tongue mobility in 1052 subjects.' *Sleep Breath* 21, no. 3 (2017): 767-775. doi: 10.1007/s11325-016-1452-7. Epub 2017 Jan 17. PMID: 28097623.

Yoon, AJ, Zaghi, S, Ha, S, Law, CS, Guilleminault, C, and Liu, SY. 'Ankyloglossia as a risk factor for maxillary hypoplasia and soft palate elongation: a functional-morphological study.' *Orthod Craniofac Res* 20, no. 4 (2017): 237-244. doi: 10.1111/ocr.12206. Epub 2017 Oct 10. PMID: 28994495.

Zaghi, S, Shamtoob, S, Peterson, C, Christianson, L, Valcu-Pinkerton, S, Peeran, Z, Fung, B, Kwok-Keung Ng, D, Jagomagi, T, Archambault, N, O'Connor, B, Winslow, K, Lano, M, Murdock, J, Morrissey, L, and Yoon, A. 'Assessment of posterior tongue mobility using lingual-palatal suction: progress toward a functional definition of ankyloglossia.' *J Oral Rehabil* 48, no. 6 (2021): 692-700. doi: 10.1111/joor.13144. Epub 2021 Jan 17. PMID: 33386612; PMCID: PMC8247966.

Zaghi, S, Valcu-Pinkerton, S, Jabara, M, Norouz-Knutsen, L, Govardhan, C, Moeller, J, Sinkus, V, Thorsen, RS, Downing, V, Camacho, M, Yoon, A, Hang, WM, Hockel, B, Guilleminault, C, and Liu, SY. 'Lingual frenuloplasty with myofunctional therapy: exploring safety and efficacy in 348 cases.' *Laryngoscope Investig Otolaryngol* 4, no. 5 (2019): 489-496. doi: 10.1002/lio2.297. PMID: 31637291; PMCID: PMC6793603.

Zicari, Anna Maria, Marzia Duse, Francesca Occasi, Valeria Luzzi, Emanuela Ortolani, Flaminia Bardanzellu, Serena Bertin, and Antonella Polimeni. 'Cephalometric pattern and nasal patency in children with primary snoring: the evidence of a direct correlation.' *PLoS One* 9, no. 10 (2014): e111675.

About the author

Dr Donny Mandrawa, BDSc (Melbourne) FICOI FPFA FIADFE PGDip Orthodontics Dentofacial Orthopedics (UK)

In 1998, Dr Donny graduated from the University of Melbourne, Australia, as a general dentist. His first exposure to orofacial myofunctional orthodontics was in 2001.

He pursued further education in the fields of dentofacial orthopedics and orthodontics by completing the mini residency programs of Dr Skip Truitt in 2002 and Dr Derek Mahony in 2005. Additionally, he gained extensive knowledge and understanding of the whole body connection, by undergoing studies in chirodontics, in 2003, from Dr Robert Walker. In 2008, he completed the mini residency program by Dr Steven Olmos, in temporomandibular joint (TMJ) dysfunctions and motor reflexes. He then obtained his Invisalign accreditation in 2010.

An opportunity came up in 2002 for him to travel to the north of India, as a dental volunteer. He was one of a group of only two dentists and two dental assistants, treating hundreds of Nepalese orphans for their acute dental needs, over a number of weeks. During his time there, he was based mainly in Dharamshala, and was fortunate enough to meet with the Dalai Lama.

In 2004, he co-founded his first dental practice in the west of Melbourne, followed by establishing his second in the east of the city, in 2012. He co-founded his third in 2017, located in the suburb of North Melbourne.

Dr Donny's interests in early intervention and myofunctional orthodontics developed intensely through the years. He learnt the art of orofacial myofunctional therapy from The Coulson Institute by Sandra Coulson (speech pathologist) on multiple occasions, along with further training from the Myofunctional Research Company. He also deepened his knowledge and skills of evaluating and managing tethered oral tissues, from the Tongue Tie Institute, by Dr Marjan Jones and Dr Dan Hanson.

With his passion for helping the future generations to become healthier, he began educating various health professionals to spread the message broadly, with his first lecturing engagement being in 2014, to an audience of 150 dentists, for the University of Airlangga in Surabaya, Indonesia.

In 2017, he began co-educating with Dr Dan Hanson, as Myofocus Education. They taught dentists, orthodontists, orofacial myologists, oral health therapists, chiropractors, osteopaths, speech pathologists, ear, nose, and throat specialists, lactation consultants, and other health providers, in-person around Australia, Japan, the US, and Malaysia, but to plenty more corners of the globe through their online educational platform. Dr Donny also presented as part of a panel of multi-disciplinary health providers in the inaugural International Consortium of Ankylofrenula Practitioners Conference in Toronto, Canada, in 2018.

Together with Dr Dan Hanson, Dr Donny co-created the Myofocus Take Off Algorithm, which is the first-ever system of delivering orofacial myofunctional therapy using individualized algorithmic prescriptions. They created 180 different prescriptions to train patients in correcting their orofacial dysfunctions.

Another medium that he uses to educate more people about holistic functional oral health is through social media. His followers on his Facebook and Instagram pages are steadily building. He shares many case studies, research papers, and interesting health concepts through them.

Dr Donny is a Fellow of the International Congress of Oral Implantology, a Fellow of the Pierre Fauchard Academy, and a Fellow of the International Academy of Dental Facial Esthetics. He has also received his Post Graduate Diploma in Orthodontics and Dentofacial Orthopedics from the London Dental Institute in the United Kingdom. As an airway-centric myofunctional dentist, he has now restricted his practice to early intervention orofacial myofunctional dentistry, within the scopes of dentofacial orthopedics, orthodontics, dental sleep medicine, and tethered oral tissues. His youngest patient so far was two days old, and his oldest was 74 years old.

As of 1st July 2025, Dr Donny is no longer running courses, seminars, and symposiums, as part of Myofocus Education. He does still guest present, on invitational bases, at scientific conferences and meetings in Australia and internationally. He is now focusing on further studies and implementing new protocols to help the future generations to receive even better functional healthcare. His passion remains at helping children with their growth and development, from a myofunctional dentistry perspective.

Instagram: @drdonnymandrawa
Facebook: @drdonnymandrawa
Web: themyofunctionalcentre.com.au

Glossary of key terms for parents

This glossary explains common terms parents may come across when learning about tongue-ties, breathing, and children's growth and development. Each term is described in simple language to help you understand what it means and why it matters.

Airway: The body's breathing passage: the route that lets air travel in and out of the lungs.

Alignment: In dentistry, this refers to how the teeth, bite, and jaws are positioned in relation to one another.

Breathing pattern: The rhythm and manner in which a person breathes: how air moves in and out of the lungs during each breath.

Carbon dioxide: A gas produced by breathing; it is essential in nature's balance to help release oxygen into cells.

Cranial system: A dynamic, interconnected system where the bones of the skull, membranes, and fluids work together in rhythm to support brain function, circulation, and overall body balance.

Diaphragm: A large, dome-shaped muscle located just below the lungs that plays a key role in breathing.

Dysfunction: When a body part or system does not work properly.

ENT (ear, nose, and throat specialist): A specialist doctor who treats problems with the ears, nose, throat, and nearby areas.

Epigenetics: How your environment and behavior can influence how your genes work, without changing the genes themselves.

Epiglottis: A small flap in the throat that closes during swallowing to stop food from entering the airway.

Facial growth: The natural development and changes in the bones, muscles, and soft tissues of the face over time, from infancy through adulthood.

Fascia: The body's internal support web: a continuous network of tissue that holds everything together and helps different parts move and function as one.

Functional breathing: Breathing that is diaphragmatic, steady, rhythmic, relaxed, and through the nose, optimizing the body's oxygenation.

Functional health: A way of viewing health that focuses on how well the body's systems work together.

Haemoglobin: The oxygen-carrying protein in red blood cells, acting like a delivery system for oxygen and a shuttle for carbon dioxide.

Inflammation: The body's natural response to injury, infection, or irritation, aimed at protecting and healing tissues.

Jaw development: How the upper and lower jaws grow and form over time.

Jaw expansion: The widening of the jaws to create more space for the tongue and teeth.

Lip seal: When the lips rest together naturally without strain, helping with breathing and swallowing.

Mouth breathing: Breathing through the mouth instead of the nose, which can affect health and facial growth.

Nasal breathing: Breathing through the nose, which filters, warms, and humidifies the air before it reaches the lungs.

Nervous system regulation: The body's ability to keep its nervous system balanced, turning responses up or down as needed for health and wellbeing.

Neurodevelopmental chiropractor: A practitioner who helps the nervous system and body develop properly, especially in children, by addressing spinal, cranial, and postural issues to improve overall function.

Nitric oxide: A natural gas in the body that helps blood flow, supports the immune system, and enables cells to communicate effectively.

Orofacial: Relating to the mouth and face.

Orofacial myofunctional therapist: A professional who teaches exercises to improve the functions and postures of the muscles of the mouth and face.

Orofacial myofunctional therapy: Exercises that help improve the functions and postures of the muscles of the mouth and face.

Parasympathetic nervous system: The part of the nervous system that helps the body rest, digest, and recover.

Posture: The way the body is held while standing, sitting, or moving.

Primitive reflexes: Natural, automatic movements babies are born with that help them survive and develop, which normally disappear as the nervous system matures.

Sleep Disordered Breathing: A condition where a person's breathing is irregular, interrupted, or reduced during sleep, which can affect oxygen levels, sleep quality, and overall health.

Sympathetic nervous system: The body's accelerator that controls involuntary body functions, activating the body to respond to stress, danger, or activity by increasing alertness, energy, and physical readiness.

Tongue posture: The position of the tongue when resting; ideally, it should sit up against the roof of the mouth.

Tongue-tie: A condition where the attachment under the tongue is restricting the tongue's range of mobility, resting posture, and functionality.

Vagus nerve: The body's main 'rest and digest' nerve, connecting the brain to many organs and helping the body stay calm, regulate digestion, and maintain internal balance.

Wound healing: The process by which the body repairs and rebuilds tissue after an injury or procedure.

This glossary is provided for general understanding and is not intended as medical advice. Always consult qualified health professionals regarding your child's care.

www.ingramcontent.com/pod-product-compliance
Lightning Source LLC
LaVergne TN
LVHW052110210926
848482LV00024B/401